OPTIMUM WEIGHT CONTROL

Know what works
Losing weight is different for everyone

Dieting is not enough
Multiple tactics are needed

Why are we the fattest people in history

What's changed?

The secrets to long-term weight loss

PUBLISHING DETAILS

Sources

Most of the evidence, data, studies and trials in Live Longest are accessed from the top medical journals and national statistics after the year 2000. Most are the latest available. National surveys and audits can cover longer time periods; but these older figures and statistics are still relevant. Some graphs used are preferred because they are the most user friendly. This information is up to date as of 2019.

Lies, Damned Lies and Statistics

This is a book for the general reader. I have tried not to saturate it with too many overwhelming and boring figures; but the references are there for the medical reader or anyone who wants more detail. Where and when the study is so huge it should convince even the greatest skeptic, I may give a number or a percentage that is relevant and reassuring- such as the finding that meditation reduced cardiovascular events by 45%, which even encouraged me to try it.

Disclaimer

This book is for information only and should not be used for any treatment without consulting and discussing it with your doctor. Opinions and techniques differ within the medical profession. The author and publisher expressly disclaim responsibility for any consequence arising from use of the information contained in this book.

ISBN-13: 978-0-9953996-6-2

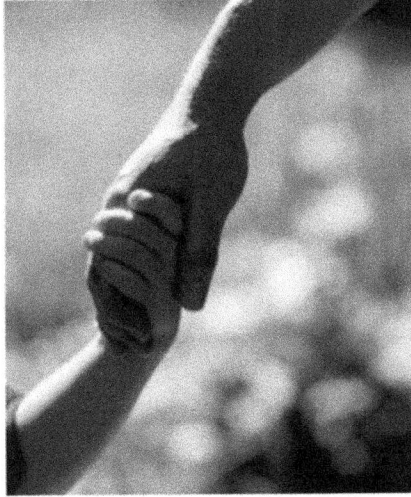

Live Longest Series:
Books for Total Health & Longevity

Book 1
The Missing Keys: Avoidance of illnesses at your age

Book 2
Nutrition: The Super-Mediterranean Diet
The foods evidenced to donate health

Book 3
Successful Ageing
Staying fit and functional from age 18

Book 4
Slim 4 Life
The best and most complete medical program

Book 5
Live Longest Compendium
Condensed essentials of Books 1 to 4.

livelongest.com.au

Now to perform a true physician's part
And show I am a perfect master of my art,
I will prescribe what diet you should use,
What food you ought to take, and what refuse.

Ovid 43 BC-17 AD

"Never eat more than you can lift."   Miss Piggy

"A gourmet is just a glutton with brains."   Philip Haberman Jr, Vogue 1961

"Matter cannot be created or destroyed but can only be changed from one form to another."   Newtons 1st Law of Thermo-Dynamics

Fad Diets and Scams have been being recycled for over 2,000 years including the Cabbage, Tapeworm, Vinegar Diets… and you name it.

Fasting Diets were recorded in 606 BC and the Keto Diet in 500 BC, Lo-Carb in 1825.

Now, however, Slim 4 Life analyses them all and provides the latest and best medical program.

CONTENTS

INTRODUCTION:
Slim 4 Life is a total program

To lose weight successfully long-term, *more than just a diet is needed* and, to deliver this, the Slim 4 Life Program uniquely combines *the 4 proven essentials* for successful long-term weight loss:
1. Diets – select the best that works for you
2. Behavior Modifications – to counter our toxic food culture
3. Nutrition – evidenced world's healthiest foods "Newtrition"
4. Exercise – a 40 second burst equal to running 45 minutes

Slim 4 Life is not just a diet, not yet another fad but a whole system based on the latest and best medical evidence and 50 years clinical experience.

A record 81.4% documented long term loss success rate is possible. Long term loss is defined as a loss of over 30lb (13.6kg) for over a year.

We are the fattest generation in history. The obesity epidemic started in the 1980s and it's fashionable to now blame our gut microbiome or genes, *but these have not changed.* What then has?

Slim 4 Life uniquely identifies just what it is that has changed and what is the root cause of this obesity crisis and our weight gain.

Research shows that no one diet suits everybody and you must find the one that works for you (included in this book). This contradicts trying a strict "Fad" diet. Incredibly
- Only 20 extra calories a day are needed to gain weight
- Only 100 extra calories a day to become obese
- But we can eat 1000 calories extra a day and not detect it

Most people have gradually, insidiously slipped into the habit of undetected overeating, but we can now un-learn.

If we can gain weight, we can lose it. It can be done. But you need the Slim 4 Life system and complete program.

MEASUREMENTS and CLASSIFICATION

> **Measuring Recommendations**
>
> Your mirror, waist circumference and weight are all you need.
>
> It's pretty obvious if we are fat or even slightly overweight...or is it? The 'Mind-Eye Gap' makes anorexics think they are fat and fat people think they are slimmer than they are – hence the mirror can lie – better get measured.

1. Weight

Weight is the simplest monitor of fat loss.

To enhance accuracy: Use digital or beam scales, measure to the nearest 100g, no shoes, same clothes (naked best), empty bladder, same time of day.

2. Height

Bare feet kept together and head horizontal (Frankfort line from lower border of eye orbit to ear canal).

3. BMI / Body Mass Index

BMI is the most used measurement today

It is your weight in kilograms divided by the square of your height in meters

$$BMI / kg/m^2 = Body\ Mass\ Index = \frac{Weight\ (kg)}{Height\ (m)^2}$$

<18.5	Underweight
18.5 – 24.9	Healthy
25 – 29.9	Overweight
30 – 39.9	Obese
>40	Morbidly obese

*   Above a BMI of 25 both illness & mortality increase

*   Optimum weight for good health and longevity is a BMI of 20 – 25

The BMI is a relatively crude measurement and not of much use in athletes or muscular people. Its main use is in population surveys. It is often criticized because it doesn't take into account gender differences and doesn't distinguish between bone mass, muscle mass and excess fat. And it requires a set of scales and a tape measure to calculate.

4.   Relative Fat Mass index (RFM)

Developed at Cedars-Sinai Medical Center, it requires just a tape measure and is claimed to be a more accurate picture of one's body fat (than BMI) and more predictive of adverse health issues (as is waist measurement itself). It involves calculating a ratio from the height and waist measurements in meters, which is multiplied by 20 before being subtracted from a figure to take into account differences for gender.

Take height and divide by waist circumference, both in meters, then multiply this by 20 and for men subtract this from 64 and for women from 76:

RFM

MEN: 64 – (20 x height/waist circumference in meters)

WOMEN: 76 – (20 x height/waist circumference meters)

Obesity: Men   > 22.8   Time to lose weight!

Women > 33.9

5.   Waist Circumference

This is the simplest and arguably the best. It gives a better prediction of visceral fat, which is the most harmful for metabolic disease risks, as well as total body fat. To avoid the complications of obesity it is essential that the following waist measurements for both sexes be achieved, regardless of height or build

Men   < 102 cm

Women < 88 cm (very bad > 95)

While it used to be measured midway between the hip crest and lower ribs a more accurate standardization is to measure placing the measuring tape around the trunk (unclothed waist) in a horizontal plane at the level of the uppermost lateral border of the right ilium (hip bone) during standing position at the end of the expiration, without holding the stomach in. The measurement was recorded to the nearest 0.1 cm.

Waist circumference should be measured midway between the lower rib margin and iliac crest (outside top of hip bone) with a horizontal tape at the end of gentle expiration and without holding the stomach in. A loss of 1 kg equates to a loss of 1 cm waist circumference.

6.   The Waist : Hip Ratio

This is no longer used much but it suggests the body 'shape' has more to do with heart problems than just obesity per se and concludes '*It is probably more important to look in the mirror than look at the scale*'.

7.   Fat % Scales / Bioimpedence

Are not worth the money. Scales that measure body bioelectrical impedance are no better than waist circumference measurement.

8.   Imaging

Magnetic Resonance Imaging (MRI) best shows visceral fat deposits, which are more responsible for metabolic abnormalities, but these are for advanced medical studies.

9.   Bod Pod

Laboratory use

Target Weight   *BMI < 25*

Target Size
Men   waist   < 102 cm
Women waist   < 88 cm (certainly < 95 cm)

Waist measurements over the above figures reflect a direct correlation with the deposition of intra-abdominal fat, shortness of breath climbing stairs, diabetes 2, at least one major cardiovascular risk factor and difficulties in everyday activities. There are more people exceeding these waist measurements than having a BMI>31. Slight waist reduction (5 to 10cm) can result in improvement in several cardiovascular risk factors.

Measurement Intra-Abdominal, Visceral Fat

Non-obese: Women: DEXA superior
                        Men: DEXA or waist circumference
                        measure equally well
MRI superior to all

DEFINITION: OVERWEIGHT AND OBESITY

Overweight and obesity are defined as abnormal or excessive fat accumulation that presents a risk to health, according to both the Centers for Disease Control and the World Health Organization. It is a disorder of energy (calorie) balance where Calories ingested exceed Calories burnt off.

Obesity is categorized by BMI > 30 and is reflected by an increased waist circumference.

NOMENCLATURE: Calories or Kilojoules
Scientists are forever changing names. This often has a valid reason but sometimes it flies in the face of common sense such as when 'High in calories' is now 'Energy dense' and good nutrition is now 'Nutrient dense'. We also have to keep converting kilojoules back to calories. We have all worked with calories and that is the nomenclature I shall use along with High or Good nutrition.
Calories were originally Kilocalories and the abbreviation was Cals (capital "C"). In this age let's go with the flow – Cals or cals, we all know what they mean.

AVOID FOOD BLOGGERS
At the European Conference on Obesity (ECO) 2019, it was presented how nine leading UK weight management blogs were assessed with only one being trustworthy. It was the only one run by an accredited nutritionist whereas most bloggers had no relevant qualifications and their blogs lacked credibility and included unhealthy recipes.

A

CALORIES

or

GENES

CHAPTER 1

THE ELEPHANT IN THE ROOM

Think Differently and Logically

Whoops, I was not calling any person an elephant.

The *real* elephant, that no one acknowledges and pretends isn't there, is that every overweight person is *eating too much and invariably too much of the wrong foods.*

How can it possibly be otherwise?

Do you inhale fat cells? Or, when you are asleep, do the Fat Elves slip under the gap under your door and inject cellulite? Or what?

The only way to get fat, that I or medical science know, is to eat more food than we need or can burn off. But burning it off is not efficient.

While it is now medically 'fashionable' to blame our genes and gut microbiome, they have not changed yet we are witnessing a new epidemic of Obesity. This was only first noticed in the 1980s, some 20 years after WW2 and following the invention spurt and mass marketing of processed foods.
Only the food, and amount we eat has changed, *not* our genes or gut flora.

That said, genes do play a part in some 6% 0f the population:

A recent study[1] (published April 2019) of 500,000 people found 6% of European-ancestry individuals in the general United Kingdom population carry a genetic alteration that mutes appetite. These people had been thin all their lives, and not because they had unusual metabolisms. They just did not care much about food. They never ate enormous amounts, never obsessed on the next meal and had greatly reduced rates of diabetes and heart disease.

A second study in the same journal[2] also used data from this population to develop

---

[1] Cell: DOI:https://doi.org/10.1016/j.cell.2019.03.044
[2] Cell: DOI:https://doi.org/10.1016/j.cell.2019.03.028

a genetic risk score for obesity. It can help predict, as early as childhood, who is at high risk for a lifetime of obesity and who is not.

Together, these studies confirm that there are biological reasons that some people struggle mightily with their weight while others do not. People who gain too much weight or fight to stay thin feel hungrier than naturally thin people.

But that, it would seem, is just 6% of us.

This is not a book for the medically obese, nor for this 6%, but, as stated elsewhere, it is for those of us who were once slim but have now insidiously put on weight and are having difficulties taking it off.

Maybe that's 94% of us!

Overweight and Obesity
This **Slim 4 Life Program** is only for the Overweight. There is a difference between Overweight and Obese. When we are overweight our control mechanisms may be able to be re-set but with obesity these regulatory mechanisms may have been permanently re-set.

Weight   = Food intake minus exercise
or, more accurately,

Fat   = Food Type (Processed Junk) minus exercise
And exercise doesn't lose much (but is essential).

Food   = 85%

Exercise = 15%

The Irrefutable Law of Physics and Weight Loss
The body cannot put on weight unless it gets it from food.

Newtons 1st Law of Thermo-Dynamics states *"Matter cannot be created or destroyed but can only be changed from one form to another"*.

Or, we cannot create matter or fat out of thin air, we can only convert it from one form, i.e. food, into another, into energy (calories) to drive our body systems metabolic needs. If, however, we eat more than our metabolic needs food then converts into fat.

Excess Food = Fat Excess

Or "calories in-calories out": If you overeat you gain weight; if you under-eat you lose. See the back cover: Eat less calories and you lose weight!

Slim 4 Life, however, is a whole Program and not just calorie reduction.

As the Definition pointed out, Overweight *"is a disorder of energy (calorie) balance where Calories ingested exceed Calories burnt off"*. Most calories are burned off running our body systems and functions while exercise only burns of 15%. You cannot gain weight unless excess calories for our metabolic needs are eaten. "Matter" (fat) cannot be created.

Different food groups, (Protein, Carbs, Fat) have different amounts of calories per gram, which allows us to eat those lower in calories

There are some of us who are genetically programmed to gain weight and who pile it on, while there are others who are 'naturally skinny'. But we will cross that.

While there is no one diet that works for everyone" there is a *key that, in fact, does 'work for everyone' – across all successful weigh loss diets.*

All weight loss diets depend, one way or another, on you eating less. Their success depends on either fooling you by some strict regime, printed menus or calorie controlled prepared meals, and, the stricter the better: We like to be disciplined and told what to do – that way we can blame someone else and try another diet when this one fails.

But hand in hand are today's labor-saving devices, sedentary lifestyles and fast-food.
- We are not all created equal and one person can eat a kilogram of food and will put on a kilogram while another will hardly gain any weight. This is due both to genetics and our gut flora (microbes)
- We can blame our genes, we can blame our gut microbiome but we can't alter these and they were here before this obesity epidemic, whereas processed food in excess was not. The only way, if we are to lose weight,

is we have to eat less calories and avoid processed foods
- Even when gastric bypass or sleeve surgery is performed for obese patients, they only lose weight because they *now eat less*.

The Bottom Line then is, how to get you to match your intake with your metabolic needs. **Slim 4 Life** not only provides the practical system and plan but at the same time you will learn about nutrition and how our bodies control weight for a life-long acceptable beneficial Lifestyle

METABOLISM
Our Resting (RBR) or Basal Metabolic Rate (BMR) is the energy we expend running our bodies and while we may think our heart and muscles need most energy it is, in fact, our liver and brain.

Basal Energy Expenditure Breakdown
This is where your calories go: 75% of Calories are spent on our BMR
> Liver 27%
> Brain 19%
> Skeletal Muscle18%
> Kidneys 10%
> Heart 7%
> Other organs 19% e.g. keeping our blood at 36.8°C.

This BMR keeps the body in 'homeostasis' and we need only eat enough calories to maintain it.

You can increase this BMR by exercising your skeletal muscles i.e. exercise, but by very few other means.

So, if you eat more than this amount, you put on weight.

Daily Calorie Needs. Exceed these and gain weight.

Gender	Age (yrs)	Sedentary	Moderately Active	Active
Female	4-8 9-13 14-18 19-30 31-50 51+	1,200 1,600 1,800 2,000 1,800 1,600	1,400-1,600 1,600-2,000 2,000 2,000-2,200 2,000 1,800	1,400-1,800 1,800-2,200 2,400 2,400 2,200 2,000-2,200
Male	4-8 9-13 14-18 19-30 31-50 51+	1,400 1,800 2,200 2,400 2,200 2,000	1,400-1,600 1,800-2,200 2,400-2,800 2,600-2,800 2,400-2,600 2,200-2,400	1,600-2,000 2,000-2,600 2,800-3,200 3,000 2,800-3,000 2,400-2,800

More specific estimates appropriate to your height are available on the Internet

Unfortunately, if you lose a great amount of fat the BMR falls and now you have to eat even less. This is why the Biggest Losers put it back on. To lose weight long term this is to be avoided

Attempting to lose weight is a biological challenge as the body systems are geared to homeostasis or keeping our weight steady:
Calories In = Calories needed to maintain our metabolism / body functions

The Overweight-Obesity Epidemic
Obesity was only noticed to be a problem in the 1980s. It is fashionable to blame our genes or our gut microbiome, *but these have not changed*. So, what is the cause?

Food Glorious Food
We are programmed to eat, and we love it. "If you don't eat you die". Every day we are assaulted, tempted, seduced, allured, enticed or invited to eat and to eat incredibly bigger portions than previously. But, in addition and most sinisterly, our food has changed more in the last 60 years than the previous 60,000.

Since WW2, over 85,000 new, often non-tested chemicals have been invented and many have entered our food chain. And these processed foods are available in excess, 24 hours a day, seven days a week, home delivered, or drive thru and they taste delicious. In fact, the Commercial Food Industry employs the smartest scientists just to produce a "product" that hits our "bliss point". Yum, yum, overfill your tum. Unfortunately, we don't seem able to metabolize this new processed "food" of refined carbs, saturated fats and additives.

Processed Cascade

The problem with foods that make people fat isn't all caused in that they have too many calories, but also, it's that they cause a cascade of reactions in the body that promote fat storage and make people overeat. Processed carbohydrates—foods like chips, sugar-soda/soft drinks, crackers/cakes/biscuits, and even white rice—digest quickly into sugar and increase levels of the hormone insulin.

> ## IF IT TASTES LIKE BLISS
> ## GIVE IT A MISS

Home Cooking

Women have entered the workforce and there is "no little wife at home to cook meals" and with modern day work, the pace of life and the distractions of modern life, we don't have the time to cook and the really attractive Supermarket package and TV advertisements says its contents are healthy, natural, enriched, lite, no cholesterol, all your daily vitamins and more. And it's so easy just to get a pizza or some Thai food and some ice cream and a cola home delivered.

Cheaper

These Fast Foods are three times cheaper than healthy foods which, of course, penalizes the poor.

Altered Tastes

Modern foods have been vastly altered from their original. Cattle no longer graze on grass, chooks no longer pick on pastures and much fish is farmed or full of mercury. Students, who may become affluent later, are traditionally poor and can't cook so they self-select for the Fast Food Chains. We now have a generation who have never tasted natural grass-fed meat or poultry. Instead they have fed on a factory composition of artificial flavorings and additives to make it "tasty". While this may be unavoidable the long-term downside is that these kids tastes expect this over spiced artificial food and they don't even like the natural food.

It takes a long time to rehabilitate such an artificially stimulated palate to recognize and appreciate natural food.

Nutrition

The cause of overweight is overeating and, in the case of humans and Russian circus lions (true, see later), is eating the wrong processed foods.

All Diets Work

Everyone *can* lose weight in the short term but not everyone *will* lose weight, let alone lose it long-term.

All the Fad Diets or the current craze have been done before: Most are scams and up to 98% fail. It can be shown, however, that long term weight loss is possible in over 81% people. You just have to know how.

No One Diet Works for Everyone

So, the diet that works for you has to be found and it should be simple without the any exclusions or restrictions (well just one).

Mental Commitment

One essential key is your mental attitude. It is absolutely useless for you to try this unless and until you 'get your head on straight', get rid of all excuses, family catastrophes, stresses or what-have-you, and be absolutely "Determined, Dedicated, Disciplined and Resolved". No diet will work unless you have the determination.

Marathon

To lose weight it is like starting to train for a marathon or learning to play a musical instrument. These are not achieved quickly but by dedicated practice and training every day and not dropping out. Plan your campaign.

Yo-Yo

If you continue to eat as you have, dithering and dickering with different fad diets, you will continue to 'yo-yo,'.

Lifestyle

To lose weight you are going to have to change your habits, look after yourself and eat better. In fact, the best!

Genes

More are being discovered that make one person more prone to gain weight. But you still can lose weight!

Slim 4 Life, using the best medical research and 50 years clinical experience, provides a *unique total 4 system*:

1. **Diet**
2. **Behavior**
3. **Nutrition**
4. **Exercise**

Successfully take it off and keep it off

Alternative Weigh Loss Regimes

One of the best-known weight loss clinics is on the shores of Lake Constance in Switzerland. It charges *"from"* £2,300 ($4,300) as at February 2019, to starve you, allowing no more than 250 calories worth of vegetable broth and juice a day, for a minimum of 10 days.

The air fares and such are, of course, extra.

At 250 calories a day you will lose weight. But then, you will also probably put it all back on. Nevertheless, people flock there, and they get repeat custom (well they have to lose it again).

There is a strong element of masochism in such dieters. They love to be disciplined.

If you don't have lazy $5,000 you can self-flagellate by going on the latest Fad diet like the Keto or Paleo or eat what is left on the floor of the cockatoo's cage. And you will also lose weight.

And you will also put it back on.

These super-restrictive diets are unnatural. Humans evolved to eat an all-round selection of foods and not some crazy ratio of carbs to fats to protein or no grains or no dairy or no fish or what's the next scam? You can also join a gym, run and work out, but exercise, although essential, for reasons to be explained, does not lose much weight.

To lose weight permanently you need more than a diet and exercise. It requires identifying the causes of this obesity epidemic then a multiple plan of diet, nutrition, exercise and lifestyle.

CHAPTER 2

CAN IT BE DONE: THE GOOD NEWS

Slim 4 Life has conducted extensive research.

Studies show that there are different ways to achieve long term weight loss. This contradicts Fad diets as the way to lose weight. **Slim 4 Life** takes these into account to have developed the most advanced Weight Loss Total Program.

How Much Weight Is Regained

It is an inaccurate and depressing rumour that if you lose weight, 95% to 98% is regained. This is not so.

This rumor began in 1959 and was that 95% of people regain any weight they lost by dieting. This number, however, was first suggested in a clinical study of only 100 people. But the finding, however, has been repeated so often that it came to be regarded as fact.

More Accurate What Can You Lose and Regain[1]

A more accurate statistic is that most people cycle and regain weight, and those who lose most are most likely to keep it off. (The medical records of 177,743 obese patients who had no medical conditions associated with unintentional weight loss and who had been having annual body mass index (BMI) measurements for five years or longer were studied).

Patients who lost more weight early on were more likely to continue to lose weight over time. Most patients in each group experienced weight cycling or weight regain. The high weight-loss group had the lowest proportion of cyclers with 58.3 percent, while 71.5 percent of the modest weight loss group and 74.1 percent of the moderate weight loss group were cyclers.

Classification

	Loss	Weight Regained
Modest:	5% - 10%	40%
Moderate:	10% - 15%	35.9%
High:	>15%	18.6%

or

Modest losers were:	60.0% long term successful
Moderate losers were:	64.1% long term successful
High losers were:	*81.4% long term successful*

Encouragement

These 81.4% best success rate figures are far better than the previously alleged 95% - 98% failure rate. What is more, for those just overweight the results may be even better as the patients in this study were identified as *obese* and not just overweight. So, for those overweight the success rate should be even higher. But see Update at end of chapter.

Mind Games

To successfully lose weight you must change your behavior to become a responsible Mindful Eater. This sounds off-putting but really it means understanding our metabolism to balance calories in against calories out, and to not eat more than their body can metabolize and identifying Triggers that unconsciously stimulate us to eat and Habit Eating and replacing these with better habits and Lifestyle. It's more a wake-up call than a huge change.

THE MOST REVEALING AND ENCOURAGING RESEARCH:
The National Weight Control Registry, Brown's University, USA
Can It Be Done

The National Weight Control Registry (NWCR) has over 10,000 people from all over the USA with an average loss of 66lb (30kg), most of whom have kept it off for more than five years.

Long Term Weight Loss

Is defined as a loss of over 30lb for over a year.

How

Everyone lost weight in different ways

No two people lost weight in quite the same way

45% used their own programs / diets

55% used structured diets

Most had to try different diets before they found one that worked.

Most had failed "several times" before.

98% modified their diet – most cutting down their daily intake

94% increased their exercise – mostly walking

Most

Ate breakfast*

Weighed at least once a week*

Exercised one hour a day*

Watched less than 10hrs TV a week

Attitudes and Behaviors

Most did not consider themselves obsessive super-planners

Most did not think they were stickers to diets

Most were morning people

Most were highly motivated

Most kept trying different methods until finding the one to work

Motivation

More than just a slimmer waist

Health scare

Desire to live a longer life

Desire to spend more time with loved ones

Goals

Overall goal rather than a predetermined weight

Most people envisioned a loss three times greater than their doctor

Get real - recalibrate expectations – 5 to 10% is great for health

Genes

There have been 10 genes now linked to weight gain (more now)

But only 3% related to obesity

In any event they existed prior to this obesity epidemic

It was considered unlikely that successful losers were genetically
endowed or had a personality that made weight loss easier

Carrying the high-risk gene shouldn't prevent weight loss

Variables

Identify problem issues

Psychological

Logistical

Food

*Push Through the Bad Days**
*Microbiome**

Peoples' gut bacteria digest food differently and their Blood Glucose levels to the same food can rise differently. Avoid commercial cons or probiotics. If interested do your own BG one hour after food and see which food cause it to rise most and avoid or reduce

*Slim 4 Life Update

The latest research has found that

- People who missed breakfast weighed less
- People who weigh more frequently lose more weight. Weigh daily.
- Physiological testing has found that 40 seconds of SIT (Sitting Intensive Training) is the equivalent of 45 minutes of running.
- Don't push yourself too far. Have a break and an indulgence.
- There are commercial 'test kit' that claim to analyze individual reactions (elevation of blood glucose) in response to different foods while others claim probiotics alter the microbiome for the better. Both are considered scams.
- In an obesity Melbourne trial[3] both gradual weight loss and rapid weight loss participants who completed the study 71·2% had regained most of their lost weight.
- This means that while 81.4% long term weight loss is possible it is going to be hard and require Determination and Resolve.

---

[3] Lancet Diabetes Endocrinol. 2014 Dec;2(12):954-62.

B

BEGIN

CHAPTER 3

LET'S START

"The journey of a thousand miles begins with one step". **Lao Tzu**

Overview
The following are expanded in the detailed chapters.

COMMITMENT

- This is probably the most important step
- Do **_not_** start unless this time you are: Dedicated, Determined, Devoted, Disciplined, Restrained and Resolved.

and can

- Commit all the necessary time to ensuring you are successful
- Is this the time?
- Can you, and will you?
- You have to be absolutely resolved – this time!
- Can you now stick to it?
- Do not take this lightly!
- Go away and think. Are you ready? Can you get rid of all excuses which have caused you to fail in the past
- Make up your mind
- Plan. You would not just buy a keyboard or a guitar without making some sort of a plan and commitment. Think of it as starting to run or swim to get fit – it will be some time before you will run a marathon or swim long distances but start now! Train and record daily - have a plan.

Motivation

- Identify your reasons for losing weight. (See list)
- Set goals - be realistic - know optimum rate of loss.
  - We cannot all be Miss or Mr(s) Universe
  - But *any* weight loss improves your health
- Being unhappy with being overweight won't help you.

Allocate Start Time

- Ensure no excuses, no interfering social obligations

Gather information
- Desirable realistic weight
- Kitchen scales
- Smart phone app: Calorie Counter
- Suitable Exercise: SIT best – Stationary exercise bike.
  Light weights
- Recognize and Identify difficult times (weekends etc - see)

Support
- Find a person who will provide support. Inform your house-hold, partner, house-mates and ask their help/cooperation

Short Term
- Fix on short-term goals and happiness:
- One day at a time, like AA: "Just today I will eat better"
- Deal with or avoid problem situations eg weekends, take-aways

Long Term
- Long term plan - lose at same rate gained
- Acceptance of personal responsibility
- Stick to the plan and goals: Don't give up after bad days.
- Push through. Immediate resumption if lapse
- Set aside time for reflection, planning and re-motivation

Food
- Identify those foods you can't resist, and which put on weight.
- Adopt the NEWTRITION Super-Mediterranean Foods and realize you will be now be eating the best. You should feel liberated and enthused by this and not depressed, deprived or sacrificial

Plan

Firstly, count your calories for one week.

Don't panic - it's not forever! You will soon not have to. Identify Danger Times. However, people lost more with the recent Smart Phone Apps that record food intake and the more recorded the greater the loss.

Secondly, Measure

Take your weight daily and waist size say once a week or month, after you start to diet.

For goodness sakes, isn't this the whole idea? If you were a runner or a swimmer wouldn't you time yourself to see if you were improving or achieving your goals? And wouldn't you do this after each training session?

- Weight daily
- Waist monthly
- Height if doing BMI (not necessary)

Third, Nutrition

You have to know what are good foods that don't put on fat or, just as importantly, the bad foods, that do.

- Read Newtrition Foods chapter
- Select foods from the five 20% groups
- Get rid of all processed junk food in cupboards, fridge
- Ensure high quality produce
- Put fruit bowl on kitchen bench (and nothing else)

Taste Rehabilitation

As pointed out in the previous chapter, many of us have become accustomed to the tastes of commercial Fast Foods – they are delicious!

But we now have to develop a palate for natural foods. Everyone can taste the difference between an optimally ripe peach and a floury one taken out of months of cold storage. Now we have to actively seek out fresh produce and think about what we are eating.

Fourth, Triggers

You have to identify what stimulates you to eat which then become habits – which you will now have to replace with better habits.

Identify and Make alternate plans (exercise / work / hobby)

Fifth, Diet Trial

Find a diet that you can stick to: Do trials (you can mix them up). You don't fail – the diet does. All diets work, short term. Now find foods and a lifestyle that you can automatically follow without feeling a sacrificial martyr, or instituting changes you don't like being imposed on you or having certain food restrictions

- Daily Physiological (non-hungry) reduction or
- Intermittent Fasting

Optimum Fat Loss Is Achieved By:

1. Gradual acceptable, pleasant changes. Substitute good food for bad
2. Daily 20% - 25% reduction in food intake (300 – 500 cal) per day.
3. Or Intermittent Fasting: 500 - 800cals bi-weekly
4. Stress control (no snacks after a bad day). Find other outlets.
5. Determination, Discipline, Dedication, Devotion, Resolve, Restraint
6. Exclusive obsession until this becomes your new Lifestyle

7. Diary, meticulous recording twice a day phone App.
8. Get someone else to check you one day. Unfortunately, research has found, we are all prone to unrecorded snacks. But try and be meticulous. It is often this 'insensible snacking' that puts on the 'hidden calories' and this is essential to lose weight.
9. Supervision and encouragement
10. Weight loss becomes harder the longer on a diet as Resting Basal Metabolic Rate falls resisting any loss
11. Disillusionment will strike, and you will want to quit
12. You must have an anti-disillusionment plan
    a. List reasons you want to lose
    b. Have realistic goals (250g a week)
    c. Update regularly
    d. Look at your list when disillusionment hits
    e. Organize a plan and support and start again
13. Be positive for any achievement. If not losing, if exercising you have less fat, more muscle and are fitter
14. Weigh daily. Immediately try harder if any gain
15. If you put on any weight you get straight back on your diet (starve) until you lose it.
16. Exercise: SIT (best) or HIIT or 100 steps / min. Heart Rate (HR) not to exceed 40- 65% of maximum HR or HIIT
17. Resistance Training: one area once a week

Realistic Goals

It is essential that you do not have unreal expectations but have realistic, achievable goals.

Research (see later) identifies "Looking better" as our main motivation while "Health" is fourth – but the National Weight Control Registry (NWCR), finds health is an important motivator.

Surprisingly small weight losses of just 5% to 10% achieved over three to six months can have fantastic health benefits.

Most weight gain has been caused by just eating 20 more Calories a day over a long time. Most obese people eat 100 Calories a day more than they need thus gaining 5 kg a year. These are *not* big amounts and are easily brought back – if you monitor yourself. However, if you *cut back by 500 – 600 Cals a day you will lose 0.5 kg a week*. Don't cut back any more as this will trigger hunger as distinct from the deliberate 2 days of fasting. A 0.25 kg loss a week is arguably even better as this is the rate you put it on. This is optimum weight loss. This is realistic. And this is what you should aim to do.

Unfortunately, we can eat an extra 1,000 calories a day but not notice it and now it has now recorded that Americans are eating 788 more calories a day.

Most people want a fad diet because it disciplines them not to eat this or that. These Fads lay down strict 'rules' and even menus. People like being disciplined – it takes responsibility away from them. Then, when it fails, it was the diets fault not theirs and these are the people who "yo-yo" - lose-gain, lose-gain.

Rate of Loss
While it may be possible to lose more than a couple of pounds or a kilogram of fat per month this requires drastic measures and, as below, any such big initial loss is usually due to fluid loss, not fat. And even with fat loss there is invariably rebound and relapse. It is physiologically optimum to lose 250g a week or a kilogram of fat per month. If more is lost it is usually only fluid or so severe it causes a rebound.

Aim:
Lose a kilo per month but make this a kilo of fat. Finally, to end up as someone who eats well and sensibly.

Fat vs Fluid Loss[4]
The optimum rate is to lose a kilogram of fat per month. The maximum rate found for fat oxidation during exercise, in this case in cyclists, was 0.7 g/min. This means the weight changes we experience when we start exercising are not based on fat loss, but mainly on fluid loss. This is why the majority of 'miracle' diets and slimming programs produce a 'rebound' effect due to the recovery of the lost fluid. Real weight change, based on the oxidation of fat through exercise (and diet) causes a real loss of 200–300 g per week, a little over 1 kg per month.

A loss of 0.55 to 0.66 pounds or 250 to 300 grams a week is physiologically, or naturally, optimum. This is some 27 to 34 pounds or 13 to 16 kg a year.

---

[4] Acute p-synephrine ingestion increases fat oxidation rate during exercise. *British Journal of Clinical Pharmacology*, 2016; 82 (2): 362 DOI: 10.1111/bcp.12952

This should be the aim: to lose 2 pounds or a kilo per month, but a kilo of fat, not fluid or muscle.

Would you be happy gaining 30 pounds or 15 kg a year?

Yet this is the rate we insidiously put it on.

So, be happy! This is the rate to best take it off for long term, permanent results.

How to best achieve this is the problem.

God how I wish I had your willpower

As the old joke goes, when the Homeless person pleads for a handout from the Dowager in mink, saying how he '*hasn't eaten for days*', she congratulates him saying, '*God how I wish I had your willpower*'.

You only need an extra
      20   Calories a day to gain weight

&   100 Calories a day to become obese

Who Can Lose Weight

To be practical, only people who had normal range weight and figures in their teens and twenties but who are now slightly overweight which, in effect, means those with a BMI of < 30 or thereabouts. These people are those who have insidiously progressively overeaten but who may now be able to pull back to their previous figures.

People who are obese either have the genes that promote obesity or are too set in their ways to alter their bad habits.

A 2019 study by Cambridge University focused on healthy adults with a low body mass index (BMI), revealed the impact of genetics on body size is greater than previously thought. Approximately three quarters of people in this cohort had a family history of being thin. Meanwhile comparison against 1,985 severely obese participants discovered additional genes connected with poor weight control, a finding which shows "the genetic dice are loaded against them".[5]

When I first started my medical practice, I had a very fit guy who 'looked after himself' better than anyone I had then encountered, and his wife told me he

---

[5] Genetic architecture of human thinness compared to severe obesity PLOS, Published: January 24, 2019https://doi.org/10.1371/journal.pgen.1007603

weighed himself every day and if he had put on *any* weight, he would immediately starve until he lost it. That was 50 years ago! He was ahead of his time without any medical knowledge – just common sense, discipline and pride in his appearance.

Alone, Alone, All, All Alone

What this means is that losing weight is something you are going to have to do for yourself...the Government is not going to help you. For every $1 a Government may spend on health education, the Fast Food Industry probably spends $10,000 even $100,000 or more.

This means you are going to have to do it by yourself. Of course, you can get support from your partner or family, which is almost essential and good advice from your doctor or a nutritionist but, essentially, it is up to you.

The "Weight Loss Industry" has opened he gate for the plethora of Fad Diets of varying standards. There are at least over 100 currently available and most work-short term and by imposing their restrictive, often odd, menus.

By contrast, **Slim 4 Life** *is a total system* based on proven medical research.

IT'S NOT WHAT YOU'RE EATING

IT'S WHAT'S EATING YOU

CHAPTER 4

WHAT TYPE OF EATER ARE YOU

A study divided overweight people into three groups as it was proposed that different people overeat for different individual reasons.

1. Hormones
2. Genes,
3. Psychology

Identifying your type helps taking avoiding actions.

1. Hedonic Feasters: *Once they start, they can't stop.*
Personalized Diet Plan: Make them feel fuller longer. Identify your problem and plan ahead to eat less, chew slowly and wait 20 minutes.
Method: High–protein (chicken, fish, meat,), Low GI Diet (beans, pasta, lentils, Basmati rice, grains, cereals). No potatoes, mostly rice, bread, vegetable curry. A trial found that with the high protein, low GI (HPLG) diet held off their hunger for almost an hour longer.
Cold potatoes are OK as the starch changes to Resistant (good) starch.

2. Constant Cravers: *A high number of genes that predispose to overweight – obesity.*
These people are hungry all the time. They prefer foods high in sugar and fat.
Method: The approach here was to use Intermittent Fasting: 600 - 800 cals x 2 days a week
Fasting days: Meats, fish, egg, vegetables (no fruit?). Must avoid carbs: bread and pasta. Eat healthy for other five days.
Test urine for ketones – this indicates that fat is being burnt off. If any carbs (sugar) have been eaten then no ketones show up on the dipstick, Ketostix.
This is regarded as the hardest diet method.
Participants lost 1lb (2.2 kg) in 2 days. Expected loss 5 lb (10.10 kg) in 3 months.

3. Emotional Eaters: *Turn to food when anxious or stressed.*
Stress causes a desire to eat more and too much extra fat can impair the body's ability to send a signal to the brain to shut off the stress response. They prefer high sugar, high fat snacks and ate almost four times as much (10 times more chocolate, three times more biscuits and twice as many crisps) as non-emotional

eaters after being subjected to the same stress.

Method: Managing emotions by group support. Low calorie diet by changing habits. Sharing diet diaries, using emailing groups, attending weight loss meetings. i.e. encourage each other to stick to their diet. Aim for a weekly goal with other people rather than a goal too far away. Minimize stress and anxiety by group support by encouragement as contrasted with non-emotional de-stressors such as running etc. Weight Watchers is arguably best for this Group.

Identify stressful circumstances and take avoiding actions – Do Something Different (DSD - see later). Don't go home and pig out. Stop feeling sorry for yourself – that doesn't help.

4. Non-Tasters

These people have reduced numbers of taste papillae on their tongues and are de-sensitized to tastes. As a result, they need highly salted, spicy and fatty foods as opposed to the Super-tasters who taste so well they don't have an appetite for many strongly flavored foods.

Recommendation: Eight weeks low-fat diet reduces the desire for fatty foods
Even two weeks on a Bland Diet resets taste sensitivity e.g:

- No salt, chili, spices
- Not tasty foods eg cauliflower, lettuce, apples and pears
- Chicken, turkey, white fish, lean beef, veal, pork, milk, processed cheese, plain yogurt
- Refined grains – white bread. Water crackers
- Lentils, chickpeas, Butter or Cannelloni beans (no salt)
- Cold: boiled eggs, potato, cottage cheese, zucchini

People who are super tasters weigh less whereas non-tasters eat junk and salt which makes them want more and they over-eat.

C.

THE BEST DIETS

CHAPTER 5

DIET SELECTION:
"WHATEVER WORKS"

Summary
There is no one diet that works for everyone. Find the one that suits *you*.

"People don't fail, diets do".

Best are Fasting, Intermittent Fasting and Eating a little less each day.

These also donate health benefits (boost immunity) whereas Fad Diets such as Keto, Paleo, altered Carbs, Fats or Protein have potential long-term problems.

There is no one diet that works for everyone. The best are presented here for you to choose from; but be wary of the latest craze and Fad.

1. **DAILY REDUCTION (Every Day-ED)**   - recommended
2. **INTERMITTENT FASTING (IF)**   - recommended
3. **LOW CARB - KETOGENIC**   - maybe
4. **VLCD (Very Low Calorie)**   -   not recommended
5. **DRUGS**   - Caveat Emptor – Buyer Beware

FASTING DIETS
Fasting Diets would seem to have the most to recommend them: Sustainable weight loss, protection from diabetes, heart disease and cancer, improved brain health, enhanced physical fitness and strength.
What is more, people prefer them.
Fasting strictly means not eating at all and perhaps just drinking water, but there are many, many variations permitted in the fasts of various religions. Here, fasting means the severe reduction in food or prolonged times between eating which, in effect, means Intermittent Fasting.

Fasting is thought to fool the body it is being starved which makes its protective immune system kick in. There's evidence these diets bolster stress resistance and combat inflammation at a cellular level. There is a metabolic switch in which, when the liver's energy stores are depleted, the body's cells start using fat for energy. This switch is a form of mild challenge to the human body that's comparable to exercise, just as running or lifting weights stresses the body in beneficial ways, the stress imposed by fasting appears to induce some similarly beneficial adaptations. Whether you're talking about physical activity or fasting, these cycles of challenge, recovery, challenge, recovery seem to optimize both function and durability of most cells.

Fasting also makes sense from an evolutionary standpoint. Continuous permanent access to food, let alone in excess, is a relatively new phenomenon in human history. Back when sustenance was harder to come by, natural selection would have favored individuals whose brains and bodies functioned well in a food-deprived state.

Intermittent fasting has been embraced by the Millennials and was the most popular diet (more than Keto) according to the International Food Information Council Foundation 2018 Food and Health Survey. Intermittent fasting incorporates brief periods of fasting with unrestricted eating. The diet can take several forms: Some followers fast for a certain number of hours each day; others eat regular meals for five days per week and restrict calories two days of the week or engage in a 24-hour fast one day per week.

Fasting is also believed to alter metabolism, allowing you to burn more calories at rest. Older research found a 48-hour period of fasting helped increase metabolism by 3.6%; another small study found a 3-day fast led to a 14% increase in metabolism. But beware that an extended fast may cause your metabolism to actually slow-down in an effort to conserve energy, which is counterproductive to weight loss as with 'The Biggest Losers'.

There's some evidence that longer fasts donate greater benefits. Research from the Longevity Institute at the University of Southern California, has found that fasting for four or five consecutive days a month may extend life and reduce disease risks. But more human data is needed. Caloric restriction lowers levels of innate immunity and inflammation, leading to increased longevity.

1.   EVERY DAY REDUCTION (ED): The DIRECT 800 DIET

This evolved from the DIRECT clinical trial involving almost 300 people in the UK. It found an intensive weight management program put type 2 diabetes into remission for 86% of patients who lost 15 kilograms (33 lbs) or more.[6]

The 800 calories, Dr Mosley of BBC TV claims, is the magic number when it comes to successful dieting. He has found that it is high enough to be manageable and sustainable but low enough to trigger a range of desirable metabolic changes. The choice you have to make is how intensively you want to do the program — i.e. how many 800-calorie days to include each week from the start, and how to adjust these as you progress.

Or, if you cut back by 500–1,000 calories per day you will lose 0.5 to 1 kg (1–2 pounds) per week, which is considered a safe rate of weight loss, although 250g is physiologically recommended.

Mosley says that for rapid weight loss, as long as it is safe for you to do it, 800 calories a day, every day, is what you should be aiming at and that you can expect to lose up to 5kg after two weeks, 9kg after four weeks and 14kg after eight weeks, most of which will be fat.

However, not everyone can or will want to stick to 800 calories a day for long. So, after a few weeks of rapid weight loss, consider switching to 800 calories twice a week. Will you still lose weight, fast? Yes, particularly if you start with the rapid weight loss approach, and then move to the 800 twice a week. The weight management program, participants had to restrict themselves to a low calorie formula diet consisting of things like health shakes and soups, limiting them to consuming 825-853 calories per day for a period of three to five months.
Stage one: Intensive blood sugar diet fasting period: An 800 calorie a day diet for eight weeks
Stage two: A more flexible 5:2 diet- intermittent fasting, eating 800 calories per day two days a week (altered from the original 5:2 concept of 500 calories for women and 600 for men).
Stage three a more gentle plan: A low carb approach based around the fundamentals of the Mediterranean diet. No calorie counting here, but less rapid

---

[6] The DIRECT Trial, Lancet: Dec 05, 2017DOI:https//doi.org/10.1016/S0140-6736(17)33102-1, or VOLUME 391, ISSUE 10120, P541-551, FEBRUARY 10,2018

and remarkable results in terms of weight loss and type 2 diabetes reversal.

Stage four: The maintenance stage: Mosley dubs this the "blood sugar diet way of life", but it essentially involves keeping up the good work in terms of sticking to a healthy diet and weight, with windows for more indulgence from time to time. Basically this stage is sensible stuff that applies to all of us- the old chestnuts of moderation and eating well most of the time reap the greatest rewards.

Variations:
a) 500 Calories a Day Less
b) 25% Less
c) Slightly Less
a)   500 calories a day less
This is based on the fact that we are all eating too much and reducing it by 500 or more calories a day has seen people lose weight. You'll need to cut back by 500–1,000 calories per day to lose 0.5 to 1 kg (1–2 pounds) per week, which is considered a safe rate of weight loss, although 250g is physiologically recommended.

b)   25% Less

> Two years of 25% calorie restriction in non-obese adults resulted in significant weight loss, with no negative effects on health or quality of life and improved Mood, Sleep Quality and Sexual Function.

c)   Slightly Less[7]

> The other proven successful way to lose weight is to reduce the daily amount you eat by 10 to 15%. As a medical student one of my wise Professors said to "leave a third of the food on the plate". This would be 33%. I felt 25% may be more achievable, but the following long-term study into the health benefits, not just the weight loss, found 10 to 15% less food was *"certainly feasible for the average person to maintain"*.

Is Eating Less Daily Better
In one trial reducing calories every day gave better results than intermittent fasting: 12lb (5.5kg vs 11.7lb (5.3kg) in six months when men eating 2,400 cals a day reduced it by 600 calories. They were also not as hungry as the 5:2 comparison. Other trials say Intermittent Fasting gave better results.
Both are good. Why not combine the two?

---

[7] Long-term calorie restriction inhibits inflammation without impairing cell-mediated immunity: A randomized controlled trial in non-obese humans. *Aging*, July 2016

You can start by eating 15% less. Calculate how many calories you are presently eating each day, be ruthlessly honest over a whole week, then reduce by 15% increasing gradually to 20 - 25% starting by deleting processed junk foods and alcohol.

"IT IS CERTAINLY FEASIBLE FOR THE AVERAGE PERSON TO MAINTAIN A 10-15 % CALORIE RESTRICTION FOR LONG-TERM WEIGHT LOSS"

Portion Control

A small six-week trial at Oxford University[8] found the dangerous Visceral Fat (see Health Chapter) is the first fat to be gained (as distinct from sub-cutaneous fat) but also the first to be lost. In comparing portion control to exercise, cutting down the amount of eating to the size of one's fist for each meal, choosing healthy foods (Newtrition) and no snacking, resulted in

- 4kg loss
- Total fat loss = 5%
- Visceral Fat loss = 14%
- Lower cholesterol and
- Lower BP
- 5cm reduction in waist circumference

Whereas exercise had no effect.

EAT, DRINK, THINK

---

[8] BBC: Trust Me I'm a Doctor

2.   INTERMITTENT FASTING (IF): 5:2

This is a less-severe regimen: consumption of approximately 500 cal/day but only for 2 days a week.

This regime has been found to be more achievable but to also have similar beneficial effects. Periodic Fasting (IF) cycles lasting 2 or more days but separated by at least a week of a normal diet, are emerging as a highly effective strategy to protect normal cells and organs from a variety of toxins and toxic conditions while increasing the death of many cancer cell types.

IF causes a decrease in blood glucose, insulin, and insulin-like growth factor 1 (IGF-1) and is accompanied by autophagy (the normal physiological process that deals with destruction and turnover of old cells for new cell formation). Recently, it has been shown that IF causes a major reduction in the levels of white blood cells followed by stem- cell-based immune system regeneration upon refeeding.

The present favorite is the 5:2 diet. This is not only a reduced intake, but the fasting would also seem to rest and reset the gut microbiome. This can be further improved by selecting the foods which further confer health and longevity benefits as well as 'Personalizing' (see below) for hormone, gene and psychological profiles. Fasting induces ketosis. Ketone metabolism has been shown to be beneficial for the brain and improve cognition in patients with mild cognitive impairment or Alzheimer's. Risks: Diabetics unless strict glucose monitoring and insulin adjustments.

Fastest Weight Loss[9]

Intermittent fasting group [5:2 diet] took less time to reach the 5% weight loss endpoint 59 days — than those on a modest daily calorie restriction, who took 73 days.

Cutting out *refined* carbs would also seem to enhance this rate.

5:2 also reduced triglyceride levels by 40% after meals,

Variations

Find which suits you but don't swap one to eat more or lapse.

a.   **2/5 for 5 days in 30**
b.   **Late Breakfast – Early Dinner**
c.   **No Breakfast 16:8**
d.   **10 Hour Regime**

---

[9] Diabetes UK Professional Conference (DUPC) 2019: Talk entitled *Intermittent fasting: weight loss and beyond.* Presented March 7, 2019

a)   Eat only two fifths of the normal daily allowance for five consecutive days out of every 30.

The average woman aged 19 – 30 needs 2,000 calories a day and two fifths would be 800 calories. Whereas the same aged average man needs 2,400 or 960 calories.

b)   Late breakfast and an early dinner

Participants in a small trial who delayed their first meal of the day by 90 minutes and brought forward their last meal by 90 minutes lost more than twice the amount of body fat after 10 weeks compared with a control group, despite not cutting down on the amount of food they consumed. By moving both meals closer to the middle of the day participants may have more closely attuned their eating times with their circadian rhythms, meaning the food metabolized better. Alternatively, the weight loss may be due to a longer fast period overnight. Also, although there were no restrictions on what participants could eat, those who changed their mealtimes ate less food than the control group.

c)   No Breakfast Regime: 16:8

If you don't eat after 8pm until midday the next day this means 8 hours of eating and 16 hours of fasting. The clue here is to miss breakfast – if you can. But don't do this if you find it difficult and makes you miserable. Breakfast has become a habit, a ritualistic reward that people feel prepares them for the horrors of the day that await!

But it is not necessary and if you can go without do so as fasting 16 hours has evidenced benefits, but a new research claims 'Breakfast Skippers face Higher CV Mortality' but an accompanying editorial cautioned against over-interpreting the observational findings, noting that causation wasn't proved. Personally, I doubt it very much indeed.

When my wife and I work we don't eat breakfast – and don't miss it. But at the weekends, with the fridge there and food on the counter we pick and pick. But even then, I've noticed we ingest smaller amounts.

And, once a month we have a treat of poached eggs on toast with rocket (arugula), tomatoes and, if we can get it, non-preservative bacon.

The occasional reward is to be welcomed, enjoyed and the longer interval, as opposed to a daily ritual, sure makes it taste better

It was a Seventh Day Adventist 'promotion' for their cereal breakfasts as per

Dr Kellogg and then the Bacon producers, to promote breakfast as *"the most important meal of the day"*. Yeah sure! Processed grains full of sugar and bacon full of preservatives implicated in bowel cancer. Why not add deep fried Hash-browns to clog your coronary arteries.

If you want and need breakfast, see "The World's Best Breakfast" in the Nutrition chapter. If not, then certainly do not feel you *"have"* to have it.

One study published January 29, 2019 in *Scientific Reports*, concludes *"Recent aging studies have shown that caloric restriction and fasting have a prolonging effect on lifespan in model animals"*.

And, also, in January 2019 *The BMJ* (British Medical Journal) published a meta-analysis that seeks to bring together the available evidence (doi:10.1136/bmj.l42) and found that people who usually eat breakfast consume on average 260 kcal a day more than those who skip breakfast and weigh on average 0.44 kg more. In other words, they find no evidence that eating breakfast helps with weight loss, and their results indicate that it might even lead to weight gain.

The editorial went on: "Prescriptive slow-moving dietary guidelines filled with erroneous information look increasingly counterproductive and detract from important health messages. The lack of high-quality evidence in this area is embarrassing, especially when dieting is a $multibillion industry, when meta-analyses of weight loss drugs include dozens of trials, and when so many guidelines recommend eating breakfast as a way to lose weight. It may be that, on the issue of whether eating breakfast is a good idea, there is no one answer for everyone. But we should really know whether that is the case".

Entitlement Trap: Because you have gone without food for so long you now gorge and overeat. If you wish to lose weight you must only have a 'normal' dinner or better still a smaller dinner.

d)   The 10 Hour Regime
Animal experiments found that restricting food intake to 10 hours a day, and fasting the rest, can lead to better health, regardless of our biological clock. Up to sixteen weeks of intermittent fasting without otherwise having to count calories helps fight obesity and other metabolic disorders. Such fasting already shows

benefits after only six weeks.[10]
Studies in animals over the past 85 years have supported the notion that calorie restriction can increase the lifespan by reducing inflammation and other chronic disease risk factors.

This is the first study to examine these effects over two years on healthy, normal, or slightly over-weight individuals and observe that caloric restriction reduces inflammation without compromising other key functions of the immune system. The test group had a significant and persistent reduction in inflammatory markers.

Our initial enthusiasm will want us to try eating 25% less but there is an inherent danger of rejection of this with relapse to our former "threshold" - the food our stomach expects to feel satisfied as well as other effects from too drastic a reduction. The best advice is to start at 10% less and when your stomach has adjusted to this new lower volume (usually six weeks) then you can try 15% and so on.

Two factors associated with higher BMI were eating more than three meals per day -- snacks were counted as extra meals -- and making supper (dinner) the largest meal of the day.[11]
That said if you self-monitor (see Phone Apps) it doesn't matter if you just have small snacks all day, rather than formal meals, as in parts of Asia, if you don't exceed your calorie limit.

Other Viable Regimes
Alternate Day Fasting (ADF)—1day of normal eating alternated with 1day complete fasting
Modified Alternate Day Fasting (mADF)—1day normal eating alternated with 1 day very low-calorie diet (about 25 percent of normal caloric intake)
2/5—Complete fasting on 2 days of the week with 5 days normal eating
1/6—Complete fasting on 1 day of the week with 6 days normal eating
Time Restricting Feeding (TRF)—Fasting for 12-20 hours per day (as a prolongation of the nighttime fast) on each day of the week. "Feeding window" of 4-12 hours. This is what the 16:8 regime is.

---

[10] Intermittent fasting promotes adipose thermogenesis and metabolic homeostasis via VEGF-mediated alternative activation of macrophage. *Cell Research*, 2017; DOI: 10.1038/cr.2017.126
[11] Loma Linda University Adventist Health Sciences Center

Find the regime that suits you and you can stick to.

While fasting would seem to boost our immunity unless it is followed up by reduced meals (calories) you will not lose weight. Do not feel because you have fasted you can now eat more.

REVIEW: RECOMMENDED DIET SELECTION ADVICE
   a)   **Reduce all meals every day by a minimum 10% up to 25%.**
or
   b)   **Do Intermittent Fasting (500 - 600 calories) two days a week**
or
   c)   **16:8 Eat for 8 hours fast for 16 hours (no breakfast)**
or
   d)   **Whichever as above that suits you**

THE SIMPLE MESSAGE

BUT THE HARDEST TO ACCOMPLISH:

"EAT SLIGHTLY LESS"

---

3.   KETOGENIC (KD) - LOW CARB – Maybe recommended
Ketogenic Diets are the present fad. They are extreme lo-carb diets where carb intake provides only 5% of energy at less than 50g per day or just three slices of bread or, in extreme cases, even less (20-30g). Fat then makes up 75% of total daily energy and protein 20%. Medically it is not recommended for children or pregnant women and certain other medical conditions.
While **Slim 4 Life** advocates lo-carb diets which eliminate *refined* carbs - processed foods the Ketogenic Diet reduces even the good carbs and is incredibly restrictive, not enjoyable, anti-social and not a long-term prospect.
As to both diabetes 1 and 2 there have simply not been enough high-quality trials to make any firm recommendations. There may well be benefits but should be done under medical supervision.
Slim 4 Life recommends discarding all simple-refined carbs but then plant-based

intermittent or everyday reduction across all food groups as per Newtrition.

The classic KD is composed primarily of fat (80-90%), with the remainder filled in with protein (8%-15%) and, to a minimal degree, carbohydrates (2%-5%). The goal is to mimic the body's state during fasting without impairing its ability for growth. By limiting the amount of carbohydrates and protein metabolized, energy is instead derived from fat within the body or consumed in the diet. As glucose levels decrease, fat-derived ketone bodies begin to take over as the body's main energy source, a metabolic state known as ketosis.

In addition to classic KD, there are three common variations of this diet:1) a medium-chain triglyceride diet, 2) a modified Atkins diet (the original Atkins is a high-protein diet, whereas the ketogenic diet is a high-fat diet), and 3) the low-glycemic-index treatment. These offer palatable options to dieters by increasing protein, decreasing fat, substituting all but non-starchy vegetable carbohydrates, and other strategies.

Low-carb diets that replace carbohydrates with protein or fat have much in common with fasting diets and are gaining widespread popularity as a health and weight loss strategy. "Ketogenic" is a term for a low-carb diet. You to get more calories from protein and fat while reducing carbohydrates.

KD was the original "diabetes diet" prescribed to type 1 diabetes patients before the advent of insulin, as this would prolong their lives as it has less of an impact on blood sugar levels. The ketogenic diet is a low-carb diet where you get only ~5% of your daily caloric intake from carbohydrates.

KD is very restrictive which is my reservation in recommending it. I simply can't be bothered measuring out 20 to 50 grams of carbs. Surely, it is just simpler to eat 300 - 500 calories a day less, of a variety of all good, health-beneficial foods as per Newtrition. But, as noted, there is not one diet that suits everybody and KD works, and it suits those people who respond to a strict, disciplined diet.

It has a long list of foods that should be limited or avoided, including:

- Grains and products made from grains (rice, wheat, rye, oats, barley, quinoa, pasta, cereal, pizza)
- Legumes and beans
- Starchy vegetables and tubers (peas, corn, potatoes, yams)
- High-carb fruits; dried fruit (bananas, apples, oranges)
- Low-fat dairy products
- Refined fats and oils; vegetable oil
- Sugar
- Alcohol

When it comes to what you can have, KD still offers an array of options, including beef, pork, poultry, fish, eggs, cheeses, avocados, olive oil, and coconut oil. Also included is a variety of non-starchy vegetables, such as salad greens, green beans, kale, and broccoli.

If not done correctly, a ketogenic diet carries important risks, including nutrient deficiencies, hypovolemia, hypokalemia, kidney stones, and gout, but these risks can be minimized with a properly formulated diet.

A 2019 study led by Salk Institute scientists suggests that high-fat diets fuel colorectal cancer growth by upsetting the balance of bile acids in the intestine and triggering a hormonal signal that lets potentially cancerous cells thrive. The findings could explain why colorectal cancer, which can take decades to develop, is being seen in younger people growing up at a time when higher-fat diets are common.[12]

In a most recent study higher-fat diets have unfavorable effects on gut microbiota, fecal metabolites and plasma proinflammatory factors. Higher-fat diet was associated with significant and potentially detrimental changes in long-chain fatty acid metabolism, resulting in higher levels of chemicals that are thought to trigger inflammation. These effects may sow the seeds for the development of metabolic disorders and cardiovascular disease, such as diabetes, heart disease, and stroke, over the longer term.[13]

WARNING: People with type 1 diabetes should not try to achieve ketosis through the ketogenic diet or otherwise. Type 1 diabetics don't have insulin, they cannot metabolize ketones and ketosis can result in an accumulation of ketone acids in their bloodstream known as ketoacidosis which can be fatal. If you are a Diabetic you must only try KD under medical supervision.

Too Low and Too High Carbs bad

A 2018 study published in *The Lancet*[14] analyzed the diets of 15,428 adults between the ages of 45 and 64 in the late 1980s. The researchers recorded the ratio of carbohydrates in each participant's diet, categorizing them as *low-carb*, *moderate-carb*, or *high-carb*. Low-carb eating was defined as getting less than 40

[12] *Cell* February 21, 2019,

[13] GUT March 2019 - Volume 68 – 3 http://dx.doi.org/10.1136/gutjnl-2018-317609

[14] Dietary carbohydrate intake and mortality: a prospective cohort study and meta-analysis. *Lancet Public Health.* 2018; 3: e419-e428

percent of your calories from carbs; high-carb diets were defined as greater than 70 percent carbs. After 25 years, the researchers followed up with the participants and recorded the mortalities. The deaths were compared with the carb intake from the initial survey.

The researchers showed a graph with a U-shaped correlation between carb intake and risk of death. In other words, those who ate at the two extremes (low-carb or high-carb) had higher risk of death compared to those who ate moderate-carb diets. (Keep in mind that correlation does not equal causation.)

But the study also found that despite the risk posed by carb-modified diets, the quality of protein and fat in the diet also played a big role in the health of participants. When eating a low-carb diet, those who focused on animal fats and proteins (e.g. red meat, chicken, cheese, bacon) had an even higher risk of mortality. On the other hand, low-carb eaters who focused on plant-based fats and proteins (e.g. nuts, avocado, soy, whole grains) had a decreased risk of mortality.

This study is observational and prone to errors in patient recall and recording and has been both supported and criticized but the essential facts would seem that the Newtrition Super-Mediterranean Foods and an all-round diet based on these, without any macro-nutrient (carbs, fat, protein) restriction or excess, plus calorie reduction – as Slim 4 Life Program advocates, is the way to go.

Many health experts in the past have also criticized low-carb diets and labeled them dangerous fads. A study, published in 2019 in the *Lancet Public Health* journal, found those with low-carb diets died an average of four years earlier than those with moderate intakes of carbohydrates.[15]

Unrefined carbs are recommended
Fruit, vegetables, grains, seeds, nuts, legumes / pulses, fiber

Fastest Results
But, to lose weight it is essential, however, to *cut out all refined (processed) carbohydrates.* This should be your first step and, usually, with best results.

---

[15] *Lancet Diabetes Endocrinol 2019. doi: 10.1016/ S2213-8587(19)30068-*

4.   VERY LOW CALORIE (SUPPLEMENT) DIET

These are proven to work (see the back cover graph). They are liquid supplements of some 800 calories which contain all the essential ingredients.

That's all you can have each day. Obviously, this should be medically supervised. I remember pioneering this in Edinburgh in the early 70s.

As an aside I was confused when one of my patients, who begged me to prescribe it, was not losing weight; but by happenstance I saw her leave the Chemist Shop with the Supplement...and go straight to the cake shop.

Even with VLCDs you cannot also eat junk.

5.   DRUGS: *"Summer All Year Round"* Caveat Emptor

As Obesity became a medical problem in the 1990s the Pharmaceutical Industry get in for a share of the $Billions to be made with some Drug Companies having a budget greater than the GDP of many countries. The recognition of Obesity as an epidemic and a disease "was hugely important in changing the market perception or even the consumers' of what obesity actually is and so Pharmaceutical Companies started making that choice of investing their money in this area of R&D of obesity".[16]

A safe and effective weight loss drug would be a fountain of gold.

Fenfluramine (Redox) of Wyeth caused fatal Pulmonary Hypertension and caused deaths in Europe but was passed by the FDA in the USA...and people died. But the Doctor who alerted the media via a TV interview, was rung by Wyeth and he, "was warned about ever speaking to the media again and if he did some very bad things would start happening to him" [17]. By 2006 Wyeth had set aside $21 billion in compensation. They were eventually taken over.

Glaxo Smith Kline then introduced one of their antidepressant 'Wellbutrin' which had a side effect of weight loss but they could not market it as such, so they primed their reps and a PR company to promote the "Happy, horny skinny drug' as it was also alleged it stimulated libido. They then paid doctors and provided them with Hawaiian and grouse shooting holidays to go on speaking tours promoting it. In 2012 GlaxoSmithKline was fined $3bn (£1.9bn) in the largest healthcare fraud

---

[16] Gustav Ando, Director, Healthcare and Pharma HIS Healthcare Group

[17] Dr Rich of Chicago

settlement in US history for promoting antidepressants and others for unapproved uses, including treatment of children and adolescents and paying kickbacks to doctors.

The last score years have seen many drugs introduced and then deleted. But the Drug companies will, as sure as tomorrow, keep trying as they seek the 'fountain of gold'.

A new weight-loss drug that directly targets middle-age spread has been developed. Slimmers taking the pills lost three times as much weight as those simply trying to diet and exercise. It is called "Lorcaserin" and has been hailed as the most effective weight-loss pill yet. It costs around AU$386 a month and works by activating the neurons in the brain that control "satiety" signaling fullness. These neurons become less efficient with age, which is believed to be a key cause of middle-age spread.

We will just have to wait and see but at $100 a week it will certainly cut down on the amount of food.

Chronic Inflammation

Chronic inflammation has been shown to create successions of destructive reactions that damage cells, thus playing a major role in the development of age-related diseases such as cancer, heart disease, and dementia. According to the Centers for Disease Control and Prevention (CDC), seven of the top 10 causes of death in 2010 were chronic diseases, with heart disease and cancer accounting for nearly 48 percent of all deaths. The CDC also reports in that same year 86 percent of all health care spending was for people with one or more chronic medical conditions.

Both overweight and poor food contribute to chronic inflammation.

New Weight Loss Treatment Approved

The FDA has approved a new nonstimulant, prescription weight loss aid — marketed as Plenity The oral hydrogel capsule, made of cellulose and citric acid, releases particles that absorb water. These gel particles help patients feel full by boosting the volume and elasticity of the contents in the stomach and small intestine. Over a third of patients in the treatment arm had gastrointestinal adverse events and other side effects.

D.

BEHAVIOR MODIFICATION

THERE'LL BE SOME CHANGES MADE

REALISTIC AIMS – BODY SHAPES

MOTIVATION

HABITS

TRIGGERS

EATING RULES

DIFFICULTIES and SIDE EFFECTS

STAYING MOTIVATED

TRAPS

MAINTENANCE OF WEIGHT LOSS

CHAPTER 6

THERE'LL BE SOME CHANGES MADE

> *"There's a change in the weather,*
> *A change in the sea,*
> *From now on,*
> *There's going to be a change in me"...*
>
> **by Benton Overstreet and Billy Higgins 1922**

Unfortunately, Behavioral Modification or Change is proven to be **_The_** most difficult part of any health program as noted in my previous "Live Longest" Books: *'Behavioral change results are overwhelmingly disappointing-even when people have complete information as to the risks and volunteer'*.

Certainly not to depress you, but to make you aware of the task ahead and hopefully to reinforce your determination, the Multiple Risk Factor Intervention Trial (MRFIT) offered 361,662 highly-motivated-to-change volunteers, free counseling, consultations and treatment for 10 years at a cost of US $180 million in 1980. But after six year 65% were still smoking, 50% had out of control blood pressure and *only a few had changed their diet*.

Can I run that past you again: These people were 'highly motivated' and volunteered and were treated by experts for free for 10 years...and *"only a few changed their diet"*.

So. Can you do it? Can you be one of the "few". Or will you be one of the majority, as above, who dropped out (and dropped dead).

Is it really worth it to you? It could well be a year before your hormones readjust so you don't feel hungry and a year of disciplined eating until you readjust your eating habits.

But that said, the only one of my older generation friends who is still functioning on all cylinders (he is 85), still goes running or swimming every day, rain, hail or sleet and confessed to me how on many, many days he felt he simply couldn't go...but forced himself. It ain't easy.

Unless you have his resolve, then stay fat and die younger than you should. I am not talking from a position of superiority here. It is hard for *all* of us until we have adopted and adapted. Until then it will be a daily battle. Just don't bother to start unless you are **Determined Dedicated, Devoted, Disciplined, Resolved and practice Restraint.**

But if you stick to it, research has found Habit-based weight-loss interventions—forming new (healthy) habits and breaking old eating habits, resulted in clinically important weight-loss maintenance at 12-month follow-up.

DIETS DON'T FAIL – RESOLVE DOES

The Most Important Key

I have not seen the following pointed out anywhere else, but it is something I urge you to now dwell on:

"LOSING WEIGHT IS ALL IN THE HEAD".

By this I mean: *You will now have to be <u>absolutely determined and resolved</u> to alter your food preferences to high nutrition foods, no junk and to adjust your intake, every day and every week from now on.*

No excuses. No feigned ignorance or innocence. No giving up.

This is the "Key" for all weigh loss **I alluded to which ensures the success of any and all diets.**

This 'key' is our brain, our mind, which has to be so made up, so completely resolved, so as to become absolutely committed to now eat more intelligently (information supplied herewith) i.e. "Mindful Eating".

I do not mean you have to be 'out-there' inflicting your new-found zealotry on all in sundry but you can quietly go about instituting and continuing your diet.

On the other hand, if you do want to make it known, it can assemble support and keep you at it.

Popular diets have not worked. Obesity is an epidemic. Fad Diets mostly concentrate on the amounts of fat, protein and carbs and food becomes the focus while we don't sit back and think of our overall lifestyle and if and how we can change it for the better.

Changing behavior is the most difficult but is the key to success. This requires motivation, determination and resolve.

Have you got it? Or do you think some fad, altering the ratios of protein, carbs or fat, some pill, unproven scams or a mystic guru will do it?

Sadly, none of them will.

The following chapters are really the practical systems and procedures to implement Behavioral Modification.

LOSING WEIGHT IS NOT EASY,

OTHERWISE WE WOULD ALL BE SLIM

Cognitive Behavior Therapy (CBT)
Cognitive behavioral therapy (CBT) is a type of psychotherapy in which negative patterns of thought about the self and the world are challenged in order to alter unwanted behavior patterns which focus on making changes and sticking to them. i.e: thinking positively. Getting rid of processed foods and eating better is only a part of this. *The big picture is to a more healthy and better Lifestyle.*

1.   Bad Habits
     Identify these (see specific Chapter) and break them.

2. Substitution

   Do Something Different (DSD) has been found the most effective habit breaker and exercise is the best DSD.

   Substitute good food for junk (fruit for cakes etc).

3. Triggers

   Get rid of all triggers (see Chapter)

   Get rid of all junk foods

4. Goal(s)

   Short Term: Think short-term, the future will take care of itself.

   Think 1kg at a time. Don't plan more than this.

   Long Term: A very realistic assessment of what you actually think you can achieve. Men often have unrealistic goals. Be conservative and, if you achieve this by one year, then based on your progress, reset this long-term goal.

5. Motivate and Monitor

   See dedicated Chapter

   Weigh daily. If you are not losing see the relevant section but, if you are honest, and wish to change, think on what you have been eating and how you can improve this. Get a Smart-Phone App and record everything.

6. Support

   Get your partner, friend, doctor or dietitian to help and

   encourage you

7. Self-Belief

   As pointed out, no one else can do this for you. Now is Big Decision Time. You have to take responsibility. Accept this and you can do it!

8. Rewards – Incentives

   I suggest you pay yourself – see later

The main practical hint for Behavior Modification is to "Do Something Different (DSD)". Exercise is one of the best substitutions for thinking about food (if you don't walk past that food shop you love and drop in for a snack). And you have to get away from where you can access food.

Restraint: The Three Factor Eating Questionnaire (TFEQ)

TFEQ is a research measure of eating behaviors which measures

   1) Eating Restraint

   2) Disinhibition

   3) Hunger

1)Restraint means trying to resist from eating by conscious determination in order to control body weight.

2)Disinhibition measures loss of control over eating, and

3)The Hunger scale shows the experience of hunger feelings and cravings for food.

Eating restraint is known to be associated with a lower amount of food intake, and the restraint increases with successful weight loss in behavior modification treatments. This means restriction of food intake is accompanied by weight loss.

Think before you eat! Gain control.

A fasting diet or a planned eating regime with no snacks removes temptation.

The contrary pattern, a decrease in eating restraint and increase in disinhibition have accordingly been found for those regaining their body weight. These types of data tell us that restraint in food intake leads to less food consumed and thus more weight loss, and that the control over food intake is crucial for weight development in programs emphasizing the participants' efforts to reduce food intake by will.[18]

Keep these in mind. Actively try and practice restraint. Do not lose control. Recognize hunger as a with-drawl symptom that you are now losing weight

Go to BED

Two reviews analyzed *all available studies* for weight loss regimes in children and adolescents, which give insight into adult weight loss problems and programs: *It was the combination of 1. behavior 2. exercise and 3. diet changes that help weight loss.* [19]

1. Behavior
2. Exercise
3. Diet

or   BED

If you are going to lose weight you will have to go to BED.

---

[18] The International Association for the Study of Obesity. obesity reviews 6, 67–85, 2005.

[19] *BMJ* 2017; 357 doi: https://doi.org/10.1136/bmj.j3029 (Published 22 June 2017) Cite this as: BMJ 2017;357:j3029

HEADS ON STRAIGHT

I apologize if my repetition is irksome, but repetition is a proven teaching reinforcement.

The Slim 4 Life Program for weight loss is no hi-fat, lo-carb, lo-fat, high carb, hi-protein, lo-protein fad-scam-gimmick diet. It is medical researched evidence. However, how to enthuse and discipline ourselves to stick to it, is the difficult part.

So, to "get our heads on straight" some truths, as above, need to be established.

Firstly, you must analyze again and reinforce why you want to lose weight. The Researched reasons are listed in a separate Chapter but, to cut to the nitty gritty, for most of us it is to look better, and we want to look better to be attractive. I fully support this. If people look after their external appearance they invariably look after their internal "appearance" and health.

Secondly, as noted, we live in a "Food Toxic, Obesogenic" environment where processed food is available 24 hours a day, seven days a week and can be home delivered. Processed food is a new phenomenon. Since World War 2 some 85,000 new chemicals have been invented and we do not know what they do. They are not tested or regulated until there is a catastrophe. But one cannot help but wonder if these chemicals are not entering our metabolic chains to help promote weight gain. In fact, as pointed out there is indeed the Processed Food Cascade in that the problem with foods that make people fat isn't all caused in that they have too many calories, but also, it's that they cause a cascade of reactions in the body that promote fat storage and make people overeat. Processed carbohydrates - foods like chips, sugar-soda/soft drinks, crackers, cakes/biscuits, and even white rice— digest quickly into sugar and increase levels of the hormone insulin.

Thirdly, most people are not liars. We simply can't know when we overeat (by as much as 1,000calories) unless we now monitor ourselves.
Studies reveal most people underestimate their intake. As fat increases recollection decreases. A person with a BMI of 30 under reports food intake by 40% and other studies report a 47% to 67% underestimating of how much we eat. Under-reporting is not due to dishonesty, fat people perceive portions as smaller than they actually are. This translates to how we see ourselves.

Fourth: The Mind-Eye-Mouth Gap: Body Image and Self Perception
> *'Oh would some power the gift give us,*
> *To see ourselves as others see us'.*   *Robbie Burns* (1759 – 1796)

We can't see ourselves as others do. Over 50 years ago a Harvard Professor told me how they assembled fat people in a room and flashed up photos or silhouettes of peoples' bodies getting them to select the body they most resembled. Even the fattest women mostly selected Marilyn Monroe.

The probability that adolescents perceived themselves as overweight or obese has declined significantly. The body mass index z-score of self-perceived overweight adolescents increased from 1.32 to 1.82. The gap between the reality and perceptions about body weight status has been expanding among adolescents: Only 21% of boys correctly perceived themselves as overweight in the recent survey: The number was higher for girls at 36%.[20]

> **PEOPLE UNDERESTIMATE THE FOOD THEY EAT**
> **BY 40 TO 67%**

People are poor judges of the amounts of food they're eating. The more people like a food, the larger their definitions of moderation. The more they like a food, the more of it they think they can eat. 'Moderation' doesn't define a clear, concrete guide.

Fifth: We put most of our energy into growing (lay down bone and muscle) until we are 18 years old. Thereafter we don't need food to grow as rapidly and we need less and less as we age and it becomes progressively harder to lose fat.

Finally, the two greatest drives for all animals, including we humans, is procreation and eating. Sex is the only drive stronger than food, but we can get food 24 hours a day. And, as I've noted, all the slim people I know "eat like birds". They always leave some food on their plate and they monitor themselves every day. One of my earliest patients weighed himself daily and if he had put on weight he then fasted

---

[20] American Journal of Preventive Medicine Source Reference: Lu, H. et al "More overweight adolescents think they are just fine: generational shift   in body weight Perceptions among adolescents in the U.S." Am J Prev Med 2015; DOI: 10.1016/j.amepre.2015.03.024.

until he lost it and that was long before IF or ED Diets were recommended.

My patient is still slim and when I had him to lunch the other day, looks even slimmer and still left food on his plate.

And so, the bottom line is that if you are going to lose weight successfully and permanently it will be the hardest thing you can attempt.

Certainly, nicotine and other drug addictions are also very hard to break but food is more subtle, more approved and more available...and so is booze. The Friday night binge has become almost an accepted ritual throughout the Western world but, apart from its other effects, alcohol is "empty calories" and even more subtle is that it is an appetite stimulant – we eat more with booze. Salt is also an appetite stimulant.

Losing weight will be a daily regime which only you can discipline yourself to achieve.

But above and beyond that "the lean live longest". I coined this phrase when I first became interested in weight loss (and my lean lunch guest is now a sprightly 86year old). There are, after all, some 2 miles of extra blood vessels in every pound of fat and this is a hell of an extra burden to place on our hearts. But, as can be seen in the Health Chapters, the Disease of Affluence – Obesity, Blood Pressure, Heart Attacks, Strokes, Hyperlipidaemia, Diabetes 2, Arthritis, Depression and more, make losing even just 5% of our present weight very beneficial.
The health benefits of correct nutrition and achieving optimum weight (defined as a BMI 20 to 25) are profound.

Weight Watchers is the best of the commercial support programs and it and Jenny Craig are up front and honest about getting you to eat less. Some, like Intermittent Fasting are just methods to get you to eat less and which I endorse as fasting makes us concentrate on eating less but also seems to boost our immune system. People have never been healthier and lived longer as when there was food rationing as in World War 1 and 2, the 1930s Dust Bowl Famines of the USA and The Cuban embargo.

These were natural disasters or Government imposed calorie restriction "diets", but you are now on your own, unless you join a group like Weight Watchers - mutual support works for those who need it.

But if you want to do it yourself it will require daily self-discipline and it will require you re-programming the amounts of food you eat.

Perhaps the observations of the lean, long-living Okinawans may be a good concept and premise for us to adopt: "Never feel full. Always leave something on your plate".

But people are not very good at accepting responsibility for their own health and we are not very good, in fact, absolutely hopeless at admitting or having the insight, that we may ever be eating too much. "Not me"! It's never "me".

But, if we can identify what, how, where and why we are eating too much we may accept that we have a self-created problem and resolve to correct it.

Changing Food in Home Essential[21]

Giving overweight people a realistic sense of the dilemma that they are in and the powerful forces they are up against -- including a genetic predisposition toward obesity and an increased susceptibility to many food cues in the environment -- may promote cognitive restraint over their eating in the short-term, but, *this message did not motivate participants to make numerous changes to the foods they surround themselves with.*

Behavior therapy is aimed at bolstering the person's internal sense of self-regulation over food intake and exercise. But research has shown that increases in self-control are not sustainable, and lost weight is often regained.

The powerful lure of foods high in fat, sugar and salt has been well-documented, and existing treatments do not do enough to ensure that foods kept in the home are permanently changed in ways that make self-control more feasible.

Just giving advice is not enough, *specific foods have to be eliminated and better substitutions made as well as preparing food differently (such as dry-bake not fry).*

---

[21] *American Journal of Clinical Nutrition* **Drexel University** Jan 2018

KEEP ONLY HEALTHY FOOD IN THE HOUSE

GET RID OF ALL JUNK & TEMPTATION

To effectively prevent weight gain, understanding the factors or behaviors underlying weight management that preceded the gain, is important. In many instances, especially with young women and men, if it is unhappiness and discontent with life. Thereafter, we insidiously just eat a little more and eat processed fast-food in response to the temptations of the toxic-obesogenic society we now live in. It will therefore be necessary to address (and reverse) these and any other life issues when you gained weight: You cannot lose weight as an unhappy comfort-food eater or someone who craves fast food.

Slim 4 Life Behavior Modification System:
1.   Plan
2.   Motivation
3.   Triggers
4.   Bad habits
5.   Danger Times and Situations
6.   Difficulties
7.   Reasons why people fail
8.   Excuses
9.   Staying Motivated
10. Not Losing Weight reasons and corrections
11. Getting rid of all Junk food in the house
12. Enlisting Help / Support
13. Hints, Tricks and Good Advice
14. Plan Meals Ahead

This systematically logically, properly and, as painlessly as possible, institutes your Behavioral Modification

Again, do not attempt or start this unless you have thought it through, got rid of the excuses that have caused you to fail previously and now have the time and determination to look after yourself. This is the Key.

But you have to be happy with the food and the regime you select. The best foods are detailed for you to select from in (D) Newtrition.

Most, if not all, of these habits are unconscious or 'Habit Eating', which we don't realize we are doing. As noted, diet resistant patients have been found to underestimate their intake by between 47% and 67%. (Get the Phone App).

It literally is "mind over matter" or to be lucidly clear "mind over fat".

It is your mind, your brain, your understanding of the amount of calories your body needs and can cope with (metabolize) and then it is up to your mind to firm up your determination and resolve, which is the key.

Gaining weight, in our affluent society, is not only ridiculously easy, it is accepted. There are more fat people than lean.

So, you are going to have to decide if and why you want to achieve your optimum weight. The reasons and motivations as to why people want to lose weight has been researched and are listed, mainly it is to look better whereas to get healthy isn't as motivating.

The problem is our behavior, lifestyle and habits. These are not necessarily bad but in our affluent society when most of us are working long and stressful hours, we often get home too tired to cook, have a drink to relax and get a pizza or some Thai Food home delivered and at the weekends its go, go, go when we relax, drink more and eat more.
Or, as a bored stay-at-home, what else is there to do?

Only a reassessment of your lifestyle and then your determination – your mindset – can alter and combat this bad, over-eating behavior, combined with the correct nutritional-dietary advice.

The Triggers and Habits (see later) as to why we over-eat should be analyzed then avoidance strategies or substitutions made.

In addition, junk, processed foods, high in calories but low in nutrition are replaced with best quality foods, high in nutrition but low in calories and, as a bonus, evidenced to provide profound health benefits.

Get all Junk food out of the house – if it ain't there you can't eat it…and this includes the ice-cream.

What also has to be found are substitutions or alternatives you like rather than eating processed foods.

You will have to eat less calories, but this is achieved by small, acceptable-to-you, substitutions until it becomes your new healthy lifestyle.

The first study in the 1990s, by Professor Barbara Rowles, found that people didn't notice an additional 400 calories added to their food and still ate the same dinner and meals as before, but more recent research has now found *we can't detect eating over 1,000 extra calories a day!*[22]

Just think on this.
It only requires 20 extra calories a day to gain weight, 100 a day to become obese but we don't know when we eat 1,000 calories more! Americans, as a nation, are eating 788 more calories a day.

Surely, surely, surely it is time to realize we have to monitor and control our intake – both quantity and quality – calories and nutrition.
This study went on to *"show that being aware of calorie intakes is important because short periods of accidental overeating can be sufficient to cause weight gain or impair weight loss. Indeed, some evidence suggests that increases in body weight during the festive period are maintained throughout the rest of the year. And may also be responsible for incremental annual increases in body weight. Similarly, overeating on a weekend can easily cancel out a strict diet that is maintained on weekdays".*

[22] A single day of mixed-macronutrient overfeeding does not elicit compensatory appetite or energy intake responses but exaggerates postprandial lipemia during the next day in healthy young men. British Journal of Nutrition https://doi.org/10.1017/S0007114519000205, January 2019 pp. 1-23

You must now think as to when and where are your Danger Times. For most of us it's the weekend but I have a colleague who used to de-stress after a hectic morning by having lunch. This is the classic de-stress-comfort-food reward syndrome. When he identified this as a danger time he went swimming instead and lost 10kg.

If you really want to lose weight, you are going to have to know what you are eating – both calories and nutritionally.

There is no magic bullet, no immediate fat shedding but you cannot continue to eat as you are and lose weight.

You must resolve and resolve and be absolutely committed and determined.

Slim 4 Life Program makes this as 'painless' as possible. The end result is that you will simply eat 'normally' and wonder how you ever ate so much and so much junk before.

We now have to:
- Commit
- Learn control
- Understand you are programmed to eat and must exert restraint
- No processed foods
- Restrict and control the media

The best techniques to achieve these will be discussed.

But the more we diet, the more we think about food and the more triggers stimulate us to eat and the more our resolve dissolves. If it's not in your cupboard or fridge you can't eat it.

CHAPTER 7

BODY SHAPES

It is obvious but seldom pointed out, that we all have different body shapes and types. Some people are short, some tall, some have "heavy" builds others naturally slight. Our genes mostly determine this.

It will be hard, if not impossible, to become a sylph-like wraith if your parents are "big-boned". It is usual for the child to inherit the features of their parents with one parent dominating. The point is that you can't change your basic shape, no more than if you are short to become tall or shrink the size of your feet.

You must therefore have realistic expectations and goals. Yes, you can optimize your looks: No, you cannot alter your basic shape.

What you have to do is *accept* there are parts of you that cannot be changed and come to terms with this and *accept it.*

Many, many women (and more men than we suspect) are unhappy with their appearance. Until you come to terms with this and concentrate on what can be changed and who and what you are, you will not be happy. We can't all look like the Hollywood pin-ups of the moment (and many of these are not so great Sunday morning with a hangover).

I am sure we have all seen the "makeovers" where a woman gets a new hair-do, make-up and clothes and is transformed from a frump into someone stylish and attractive. So start there.

Posture is all-important. Try a modeling school. Teeth are next.

Finally, if you do have an overly prominent nose or "bat" ears, even weak retracted chins, these can be fixed with plastic surgery. Breast implants and face lifts are available too and now buttock and "muscle" implants. But these or the desire to have these can be symptoms of deeper problems.

We are besieged as to what we should look like. Catwalk models verge on anorexia - "the coat hanger look". Men have gone from hairy chests to smooth and muscle bound. Buttock implants are "in". However, in a few years the "school-boy bum" will be back as will hairy chests.

In the main, we will never look like the ideal we want and, if we did, unfortunately, such personalities then want something else. This is a fundamental psychiatric problem: Optimizing our looks and appearance or minor plastic surgery is fine as is achieving optimum weight - especially as it has profound health benefits, but the pursuit of serial plastic surgery should ring alarm bells.

Finally, we all have different tastes and ideas of beauty and attractiveness.

By all means do your best but be wary of becoming obsessed with seeking perfections. Even the people we regard as the best-looking and most beautiful have hang-ups about their looks.

Accept what you are. Any modifications such as body-building or weight-loss takes years of dedication.

How Much Should You Lose: Slim 4 Life Recommendation
Physiologically and for health it is recommended to lose the fat on our abdomen: The 'fatty apron', the gut or wedge of fat that hangs over our belt, should go. This reflects Visceral Fat, the deep fat that is detrimental to our health (see the Health Chapter).
For a woman her waist should be less than 85cm while greater than 95cm brings a number of health problems.
For a man his waist should be less than 102cm.

CHAPTER 8

MOTIVATION

RESEARCHED MOTIVATIONS

1. Appearance. To look better; have more sex appeal
2. To improve self-esteem, pride, confidence
3. To feel better, have more energy
4. To be healthier and live longer
5. To have more control over one's life
6. To fit into smaller clothes
7. Personal goals – an anniversary, marriage
8. Overheard criticism
9. To get less discrimination; more pay
10. For a bet

Get Motivated

Motivation to lose weight may best be defined, as *"giving a person the reason, enthusiasm and determination, to change weight gaining to weight losing, behavior(s)"*.

Being motivated is arguably the most important key to losing weight. The Reasons why we want to lose weight are listed below but these are not quite the same as being motivated.

Why We Overeat

This is one step before the listed Motivators.

- What feelings cause you to eat
    - o Hunger
    - o Stress
    - o Depression
    - o Addiction – Binge eating
    - o Boredom
- Others
    - o Habits
    - o Availability of food especially in house
    - o Medications

- Re-set of previous normal intake levels
  - o   Chronic insidious little bit more each day
  - o   Processed foods
  - o   Obesogenic environment

Analyzing and thinking about these will help you address these stimuli.

The Most Important Key

I have not read the following anywhere else, but it is something I urge you to now dwell on:

> *"Losing weight is all in the head".*

By this I mean:

You will now have to be <u>absolutely determined and resolved</u> to alter your food preferences to high nutrition foods, no junk and to adjust your intake, every day and every week from now on.

What you have been eating is not normal. To gain weight you have had to be over-eating. Now, you have to re-adjust and get back to normal. This will take time and it's a daily discipline. But eventually this 'normal' healthy eating pattern will establish.

No excuses. Resolve, resolve, resolve and never give up.

The food you eat comes after you have made the decision to lose weight. What you have to now discover are the high nutrient low-calorie foods which also improve your health and what are the high calorie foods that not only damage your health but pile on the weight.

But ensure these are small changes acceptable to you. No violent changes. Replace cakes and biscuits with fruit or dry fruit (prunes, apricots etc), substitute soda water with fresh lime for alcohol.

Much eating is a habit; we want desert, or even breakfast, because it has always been the case. Try substituting (fruit platter instead of ice-cream etc). Gradually learn not to expect desert, try missing then going without breakfast.

By far and away, why we want to lose weight, is to look good and, not to be coy, we do so to be sexually attractive. You can call it 'pride in one's appearance' if you like, and I totally applaud this because, as I point out elsewhere, I feel a person's appearance reflects the state of their internal health such as their coronary arteries and other organs.

But, but, but! The most recent dramatic motivation, and potential success, has been the discovery that Type 2 Diabetes can be cured or placed in remission by weight loss. These patients avid (new) embracing of dieting 'surprised their health care professionals who had been previously used to failures in conventional weight loss programs'.
These dieters cited their new enthusiasm was 'their keenness to regain their health, not being labeled a Diabetic and not having to take tablets every day and fear of complications'.

There is a lesson to be learned here. Diabetes 2 is a simple condition of the body having acquired more fat than the individual's body can cope with. And you need not have a BMI > 25 as individuals can have a 'personal fat threshold'. Get tested.

However, having been appointed to the world's first Coronary Care Unit, my sad experience over 50 years, is that people have to have their heart attack before they do anything – despite my previous best efforts to provide prevention advice. And even after their heart attacks, if they live, they and these diabetics often default.

Cardiovascular Diseases (heart attacks and strokes) are our greatest cause of our being prematurely disabled or dead. Diabetes 2 from fat gain helps cause these, so why not _prevent_ these by losing weight!

While looking sexy and good may be our greatest motivators, the weight loss prevents our becoming a cardiac cripple, semi-paralyzed with an early admission to a Nursing Home or the Funeral Parlor.

Worth considering.

The Health Rewards
Those who lost between five and 10% were 22% less likely to have metabolic syndrome, a combination of conditions which increases risk of heart disease, stroke and diabetes -- three of the most lethal health problems.
Those who lost more than 20% lowered their odds by 53%. Not only will you look better, not only will you be more attractive, you will be 53% healthier!

Unfortunately, being healthier is not high on peoples' motivation list...unless they have had a heart attack or diabetes 2. Otherwise it comes in, down the above list, at number four.

Get Paid to Lose Weight

Money has been researched as one of the greatest motivators. There are a number of ways such as

- pay yourself any money saved from your food bill by eating less
- work out what you can afford and pay yourself say $100/kg lost
- spend less on booze

Plan:

* Identify good reasons for losing weight
* Set goals
* Recognize difficult times
* Recognize habits, break them and do something different DSD
* Deal with or avoid problem situations e.g. weekends
* Find a person who will provide support
* Stick to the plan and goals – don't give up after bad days
* Get a diet diary and Calorie counter and fill it in every day
* Fast 2 days /week or reduce daily intake 15- 25% of present food
* Small pleasant, acceptable-to-you, changes
* Like AA: 'just for today I won't eat that...'
* Immediate resumption if lapse
* Determination, Discipline and Resolve
* Long term plan - lose at same rate gained
* Acceptance of personal responsibility
* Select a diet/food that you know & understand, is beneficial to your total health & is gastronomically & financially acceptable
* Get rid of all junk. Get in fruit and nuts

Without any fear of contradiction, the best diet-foods are the Newtrition Super-Mediterranean Diet, evidenced to be the world's best.

THE BEST REASON
The best reason is usually your own reason at this moment

GOALS
Think about a particular time in the next few days and getting started
Think about each step to make the change
How you feel after exercise etc
Imagine one year hence: How would you like to look, feel and be doing.
How are things then different
What did you enjoy doing most compare now and then e.g. more energy, more active
Making goals more concrete: gym, losing 1kg, losing 3kg. Doing weights.
Doing SIT (see Exercise Chapter).

ATTITUDE
Successful weight loss depends on attitude. If you are not determined or happy to lose weight you will fail (again).

Stop feeling sorry for yourself. It does you no good and does not lose weight.

No one has the answer to what is the best to motivate you, let alone keep you motivated. But if you can get started and adopt new weight loss habits, they will become inculcated new behaviors as early as six weeks and you won't have the daily battle with motivation and self-control as at the start. Weight loss then becomes a self-perpetuating motivation.

You can wish you were thinner, you can try this or that diet, but unless you are motivated and determined to change your behavior - your eating habits - you need not deceive yourself again as you will not lose weight.

Rewards - the Best Motivators
Rewards are the most successful motivators whether it be love, the promise of promotion, an increase in salary, winning a bonus but, in short, getting something you want and desire.

Classification:

Research documents that the most powerful rewards are:

1.   **Love**
2.   **Power**
3.   **Money**

1. Love and Sex

Love comes in many forms but perhaps summed up as the most intense of emotions and, as Billie Holiday sang *"How close together love and hate can be"* and to that end, I remember a fat friend who, when I saw him after a few months, had trimmed down amazingly and when I asked him how he had lost so much weight? He replied, *"Try the divorce diet"*.

When you're married then you can run to fat or so it would seem. One problem with true love is that one partner may tolerate the other gaining weight 'because they love him or her' when, in fact, they should motivate their opposite to get slim and look good and be healthy.

I remember a New Yorker Cartoon of years ago, before jogging was popular: Here was a middle-aged man with a 'beer gut' jogging in a track-suit; one woman in her front yard observing him says to her neighbor over the fence *"Must have a new secretary"*.

Sexual Attraction

Sex is our most basic and most powerful instinct and motivator.
It may not be the real thing, true love, but most people put themselves out "in the market" by trying to look attractive which means, in our society, being slim or "having a good body".
So searching for a mate may be your best motivator.

Gotta look good!

2. Power

Power is a very powerful motivator and those that seek it usually go to any lengths to obtain it and if this means losing weight...

3. Money: Eat better, eat less, earn money!

Money is the most immediate and practical (available and accessible) of all rewards.

As you want and desire to lose weight and money is the best available motivator, why not combine the two?

If you presently spend say $100 a week on food, analyze what junk food you currently eat is most likely to put on weight and see if you can cut this down (or out) by $10 a week.

You are now, effectively, saving $10 a week and eating less junk. In the long term this translates to losing weight and this $10 a week you are now saving should be put into a separate "Weight Loss Account" as a reward. In effect you are being rewarded to lose weight.

Get Paid to Lose

Work out what food or drink you could do without if some real catastrophe hit. It may be some expensive food or behavior, such as the Friday night binge or the not so cheap bottle of wine or the restaurant meal, let alone the Fast Food Junk binge, the chocolate or cookies, but see just what you could do without in an emergency. It would be best if it were some junk food. Soda-soft drinks are the best to cut out (sugar laden) then alcohol (empty calories).

Find out what this costs, and that saving, if and when you don't eat or drink it, will be your financial reward.

Set this aside. It can be as little as $2.50 but the more the better - within reason. $2.50 a week may be too low, and you may not find this any sort of a reward - so then find an affordable amount you recognize as a reward you would be glad to receive.

Set your own maximum achievable amount you can save to pay yourself if and when you achieve the agreed weight loss.

A can of soda-soft drink is around $2.50 so one less a day is $17.50 a week or $70 a month (and you should not be having any) and there are cheaper wines. Perhaps $10 a week may be optimum while $20 a week is over $1000 a year.

By coincidence, as I was writing this, the following study was reported:[23]

"In the randomized eight-month long Trial on Incentives for Obesity (TRIO), 161 participants paid $234 to access a 16week intensive weight loss program.

[23] Applying economic incentives to increase effectiveness of an outpatient weight loss program (TRIO) – A randomized controlled trial. *Social Science & Medicine*, 2017; 185: 63 DOI: 10.1016/j. socscimed.2017.05.030

The program required participants to attend weekly sessions at the Lifestyle Improvement and Fitness Enhancement (LIFE) Centre where they were taught skills to maintain a healthy lifestyle and encouraged to lose at least 5% of their body weight.

Participants also paid an additional $165 for the Rewards program. Participants in the intervention arm could earn monthly rewards either in cash or as a lottery ticket with a one in 10 chance of winning 10 times the cash amount if they met monthly weight loss and step goals. Additional rewards were offered for meeting 5% or 8% weight loss goals at months four and eight. The maximum possible reward value over the eight-month period was $660 if all weight loss and step goals were met. Those randomized to the control arm had their money returned and were ineligible for rewards.

At the end of month four, weight loss was more than twice as great in the Rewards arm compared with the control arm (average 3.4 kg versus 1.4 kg weight loss). At months eight and 12, weight loss remained greater (average 3.3 kg vs. 1.8 kg weight loss at month eight and 2.3 kg vs 0.8 kg weight loss at month 12). Moreover, more than three times as many Rewards arm participants achieved 5% or greater weight loss at month four, relative to control arm participants (40% vs. 12%). At month four more than twice as many hit the 5% threshold (41% vs. 21%) and the percentage with 5% or greater weight loss was still greater at month 12 (28% vs. 17%).

The average payout to participants in the Rewards arm was $225.00. After subtracting the fee to access the rewards, third party costs were $60.00 per participant. Moreover, although only 42% of participants earned more than they paid in, ~80% reported satisfaction with the rewards scheme".

It was concluded that these findings not only show the value of rewards to increase weight loss and weight loss maintenance.

So it works!

A weekly monetary reward

1. Gives you *two* Immediate positive objectives
    i. weight loss
    ii. a financial reward
2. These provide practical and weekly incentives

3. This doubly reinforces commitment and results
4. Accumulating rewards become "savings" and provide yet more on-going motivation
5. Hopefully leads to better selection of foods
6. Enforces saving

Money Reward Motivation

Try this Money Reward Motivation as it is money you "earn" by losing weight and do so saving money by cutting down of food bills.

This is not to be confused with the Reasons or Benefits for losing weight which may also be motivating.

But to make this work you have to really be serious and meticulous as to your food and drink budget before you start, then be meticulous as to how much less you are spending on food, especially junk, each week and you *must* achieve or exceed your goal.

The usual reasons to relapse will occur but the most likely will be "I'll make it up tomorrow" (after exceeding your new budget).

It has to be an everyday commitment - or stay overweight.

I can think of no more immediate, daily motivation: Save money, save on junk or excess food and get paid to lose.

Functional Imagery Training (FIT)[24]

Functional Imagery Training (FIT) is a new way of supporting behavior change. Research by the University of Plymouth on FIT for weight management, published in the International Journal of Obesity, showed that FIT led to substantially higher sustained weight loss than an active control condition.

FIT is based on two decades of research showing that mental imagery is more strongly emotionally charged than other types of thought. It uses imagery to strengthen people's motivation and confidence to achieve their goals, and teaches people how to do this for themselves, so they can stay motivated even when faced with challenges.

---

[24] University of Plymouth

FIT uses collaborative counseling techniques to help people think about their most important goals, and mental imagery exercises to strengthen desire for those goals. It teaches self-management techniques, so individuals become their own therapist and continue losing weight by themselves. FIT aims to produce a 'mindset shift' where individuals exercise or eat healthily because they want to, not because they have to. Unlike most studies, FIT provided no diet/physical activity advice or education. People were completely free in their choices and supported in what they wanted to do, not what a regimen prescribed.

Most people agree that in order to lose weight, you need to eat less and exercise more, but in many cases, people simply aren't motivated enough to heed this advice -- however much they might agree with it. So, FIT comes in with the key aim of encouraging someone to come up with their own imagery of what change might look and feel like to them, how it might be achieved and kept up, even when challenges arise.

Users of FIT lost 4.3cm more around their waist circumference in six months than Motivational Interviewing (MI) -- a technique that sees a counselor support someone to develop, highlight and verbalize their need or motivation for change, and their reasons for wanting to change. And they continued to lose weight after the intervention had finished. FIT goes one step further than MI, as it makes use of multisensory imagery to explore these changes by teaching clients how to elicit and practice motivational imagery themselves. Everyday behaviors and optional app support are used to cue imagery practice until it becomes a cognitive habit. Maximum contact time was four hours of individual consultation, and neither group received any additional dietary advice or information.

The study showed how after six months people who used the FIT intervention lost an average of 4.11kg, compared with an average of 0.74kg among the MI group. After 12 months -- six months after the intervention had finished -- the FIT group continued to lose weight, with an average of 6.44kg lost compared with 0.67kg in the MI group.

FIT starts with taking people through an exercise about a lemon. They are asked to imagine seeing it, touching it, juicing it, drinking the juice and juice accidentally squirting in their eye, to emphasize how emotional and tight to our physical sensations, imagery is. From there it is possible to encourage them to fully imagine and embrace their own goals. Not just 'imagine how good it would be to lose weight' but, for example, 'what would losing weight enable you to do that you can't do now? What would that look / sound / smell like?' and encourage them to use all of their senses.

GOALS

1. Treat comorbidities first with lifestyle modification or medications if necessary, e.g. diabetes 2

2. Decide your weight loss amount based on your motivation. (A wedding anniversary, party, interview, a bet etc)

3. The first treatment goal is to stabilize body weight. Monitor weight loss daily and waist circumference every 1-2 weeks initially to evaluate the treatment plan.

4. Set realistic calendar goals based on fat mass loss (may weigh the same but less fat more muscle) and a decrease in waist circumference rather than concentrating on body weight.

5. Modest slimming (eg, 3-5% from initial body weight) can have health benefits. A 5-10% weight loss has significant impact in reducing comorbidities.

6. Initiate obesity management with a specific area (physical activity, nutrition, or psychological aspects).

7. Communicate the risks of weight cycling after weight loss.

Finally

Read the Chapter on Portion Control.

Resolve

Resolve

Resolve

Resolve

Resolve

Resolve

Resolve

Resolve

Resolve

Resolve

Resolve

Resolve

Resolve

DON'T GIVE UP

CHAPTER 9

HABITS

IDENTIFY and BREAK

Research has found Habit-based weight-loss interventions—forming new (healthy) habits and breaking old eating habits, resulted in clinically important weight-loss maintenance at 12-month follow-up.[25]

After 12 weeks, the habit-forming and habit-breaking participants had lost an average of 3.1kg. More importantly, after 12 months of no intervention and no contact, they had lost another 2.1kg on average.

Some 67% of participants reduced their total body weight by over 5%, decreasing their overall risk for developing type two diabetes and heart disease. As well as losing weight, most participants also increased their fruit and vegetable intake and improved their mental health.

Often habitual behaviors override our best intentions.[26]

Most, if not all, of these habits are unconscious or "habit eating", which we don't realize we are doing, and the key is to identify them and replace them with non-eating habits by Doing Something Different (DSD).

If you start to snack each day when you get home from work, you'll form a habit that will then "require" you to do so in that context every day.

The key to staying a healthy weight is to reinforce healthy habits.

There are two parts:
1. Breaking old habits
2. Forming new habits

---

[25] *International Journal of Obesity* volume 43, pages 374–383 (2019)
[26] Br J Soc Psychol. 2008 Jun;47(Pt 2):245-65. Epub 2007 Aug 2.

1. Habit-breaking: Try and perform a different task every day. These tasks were focused on breaking usual routines and included things such as "drive a different way to work today", "listen to a new genre of music" or "write a short story".

2. Habit-forming: Follow a program that focused on forming habits centered around healthy lifestyle changes. Incorporate the following ten healthy tips into their daily routine, so they became second-nature.

Ten healthy habits you should form[27]

Research into Ten Top Tips was undertaken at University College London and funded by the Medical Research Council's National Prevention Research Initiative. Patients reported a greater increase in the automaticity of the target behaviors, which suggests Ten Top Tips was more effective at establishing new habits. Over the longer term (2 years), patients maintained the weight they had lost which suggests Ten Top Tips is a low-cost, low intensity option for long term weight loss.

1. Keep to a meal routine: eat at roughly the same times each day. People who succeed at long term weight loss tend to have a regular meal rhythm (avoidance of snacking and nibbling). A consistent diet regimen across the week and year also predicts subsequent long-term weight loss maintenance

2. Go for healthy fats: choose to eat healthy fats from nuts, avocado and oily fish instead of fast food. Trans-fats are <u>linked to an increased risk </u>of heart-disease

3. Walk off the weight: aim for 10,000 steps a day. Take the stairs and get off one tram stop earlier to ensure you're getting your heart rate up every day

4. Pack healthy snacks when you go out: swap crisps and biscuits for fresh fruit

5. Always look at the labels: check the fat, sugar and salt content on food labels

6. Caution with your portions: use smaller plates, and drink a glass of water and wait five minutes then check in with your hunger before going back for seconds

---

[27] Developed by Weight Concern (a UK charity)

7. Break up sitting time: decreasing sedentary time and increasing activity is linked to substantial health benefits. Time spent sedentary is related to excess weight and obesity, independent of physical activity level

8. Think about your drinks: choose water and limit fruit juice to one small glass per day

9. Focus on your food: slow down and eat while sitting at the table, not on the go. Internal cues regulating food intake (hunger/fullness signals) may not be as effective while distracted

10. Always aim for five serves of vegetables a day, whether fresh, frozen or tinned: fruit and vegetables have high nutritional quality and low energy density. Eating the recommended amount produces health benefits, including reduction in the risk of cancer and coronary heart disease.

These have resulted in significant long-term weight loss without insisting on any diet. But you now have to identify your eating habits and triggers.

Mindless Eating[20]
How aware are people of food-related decisions they make and how the environment influences these decisions? Study 1 showed that 139 people underestimated the number of food-related decisions they made—by an average of more than 221 decisions. Study 2 examined 192 people who overserved and overate 31% more food as a result of having been given an exaggerated environmental cue (such as a large bowl). Of those studied, 21% denied having eaten more, 75% attributed it to other reasons (such as hunger), and only 4% attributed it to the cue. These studies underscore two key points: First, we are aware of only a fraction of the food decisions we make. Second, we are either unaware of how our environment influences these decisions or we are unwilling to acknowledge it.

Eating on the go may make dieters overeat later on in the day. This may be because walking is a powerful form of distraction which disrupts our ability to process the impact eating has on our hunger. Or it may be because walking, even just around a corridor, can be regarded as a form of exercise which justifies overeating later on as a form of reward. (People who ate snack bars on the move ate five times more chocolate). Even though walking had the most impact, any form of distraction, including eating at our desks can lead to weight gain. When we don't fully concentrate on our meals and the process of taking in food, we fall into a trap of mindless eating where we don't track or recognize the food that has just been consumed.

Stress Eating and How to Stop It

A 2017 survey by the American Psychological Association (APA) found that money, work, crime, violence, the political climate and the future of the nation are all significant stressors for Americans, each plaguing more than half of the survey respondents and, arguably, for most Western Societies. And in a different survey the APA found that almost 40% of adults reported overeating or consuming junk food in response to stress during the prior month. And of those people, about half said they did so weekly.

The Stress Response

Chronic stress can release the hormone cortisol which can lead to increased appetite.

But just as often, food is used as a "numbing strategy" - a distraction strategy in the same way that people might use alcohol or drugs or sex or TV as ways to create a buffer between themselves and their stress.

Brain imaging research has shown that when people binge on carbohydrates and sugars, it can actually activate the pleasure centers of the brain and sugar, like heroin or cocaine, and can cause the feel-good chemical dopamine to flood the nucleus accumbens, the part of the brain responsible for pleasure and reward. Sugar can also release endogenous opioids, the body's natural painkillers, which creates a pleasant effect.

Autopilot - Mindless Eating

It is necessary to identify if it is emotional or physical hunger. Hunger feels different for everybody, but it's often accompanied by physical symptoms like a growling or empty stomach, low energy and headache. If you're craving snacks without any of these physical signs, you may simply be looking for comfort or a distraction.

If you aren't truly hungry and it is a comfort food type of response, or an attempt to manage the stress that is related to using food to soothe.

How to stop stress eating

Do Something Different (DSD): Go for a walk, get some fresh air, try meditation, call a friend — can help you avoid the draw of junk food. Drinking water may also help, since people often confuse hunger and thirst.

Long-term, getting at the root cause of your stress is more important than stopping yourself from snacking in the moment. Healthy habits like exercise, sleep and proper nutrition are all sustainable stress relievers. Emotional eating is happening because there's an emotional need that isn't being fulfilled. Feeling guilty for occasionally choosing comfort food will only add to your stress.

Mindful Eating

Mindfulness has been defined as the act of focusing attention on present-moment experiences. With respect to eating it means concentrating and paying attention to the food you are eating.

The object is to think about every mouthful or food you are putting in your mouth rather than being distracted or thinking of something else, some problem, work, TV the phone or whatever. It should make you think more about hunger and fullness cues.

It has been found that "attentive eaters" ate less than inattentive eaters.[28]

And the more people became intrigued with the TV program, the less they ate; whereas they ate more with a familiar than with a novel episode.[29]

Memory seems to play an important role in regulating appetite. When people were asked to recall the detail of what they had for lunch they ate less for an afternoon snack. And the degree of hunger felt is dictated in part by our conscious awareness—not just by how much food consumed.[30] If you deliberately memorize in detail what you have eaten you will eat less.

Mindful eating may break the link between craving for a food and actually eating it. When people practiced mindful eating, they ate less in response to their cravings, and this had a small but measurable effect on their weight.[31]

---

[28] Eating attentively: a systematic review and meta-analysis of the effect of food intake memory and awareness on eating
Eric Robinson Paul Aveyard Amanda Daley Kate Jolly Amanda LewisDeborah Lycett Suzanne Higgs *The American Journal of Clinical Nutrition*, Volume 97, Issue 4, April 2013, Pages 728–742, https://doi.org/10.3945/ajcn.112.045245 Published: 27 February 2013

[29] Front Psychol. 2015; 6: 1657.

[30] Episodic Memory and Appetite Regulation in Humans PLOS/ONE Published: December 5, 2012 https://doi.org/10.1371/journal.pone.0050707

[31] J Behav Med. 2016 Apr; 39(2): 201–213. Published online 2015 Nov 12. doi: 10.1007/s10865-015-9692-8 Effects of a mindfulness-based intervention on mindful eating, sweets consumption, and fasting glucose levels in obese adults: data from the SHINE randomized controlled trial

This, if you really do it, should be enough but meditation is also being used should you feel you need it.

With the onset of overweight and obesity came the plethora of restrictive fad diets which, although not voiced or admitted to, were thought as castigatory if not punishing but many tried these.

Depriving ourselves of enjoyable foods and exercising as a form of punishment is not sustainable and often leads to rapid cycling between weight gain and loss, or "Yo-yo" dieting and even disordered eating patterns.

To counter these diets, wherein it was found that dieting and food restriction can actually contribute to weight gain, the non-dieting movement evolved suggesting that everyone possesses the natural mechanism to ensure good nutrition and a healthy weight and promoting "intuitive eating" and "mindful eating"

Non-dieting eating styles promote:
• listening to your body
• eating when you're hungry and stopping when you're full
• eating mindfully without distractions such as television and smart phones
• moving daily for enjoyment rather than punishment
• accepting the body's natural size and shape
• removing food guilt
• ending food preoccupation by removing any form of food restriction.

Non-dieting eating styles shift the focus from weight management to health promotion and claim this encourages body acceptance in contrast to the common body dissatisfaction aspect of restrictive dieting. Body acceptance improves self-esteem, body image satisfaction, and physical and psychological well-being.

This, to me, is too wishy-washy. Sure, the sentiments are fine but to me it's going from one extreme of restrictive dieting, to the other of no dieting with similar inherent risks.

There is a middle more sensible course which the following Tips advocate. Here, "mindful" means just that - we should think about our food and not just blindly eat how and what we want. This depends on good nutrition and discipline.

A simple document titled "12 Mindful Eating Strategies"[32] is among the guides provided to participants.[33] It includes such advice as:

1. **Make eating an exclusive event.** When you eat – only eat. Give eating the attention it needs to fully enjoy your food and be mindful of every bite. Eating without distraction can help you better recognize when you are full.

2. **Check your stress level.** Eating is a common response to stress. During times of stress, you may find yourself turning to food even when you are not hungry. Try to get your mind off of food and deal with stress in other ways, perhaps a few deeps breaths or a short walk.

3. **Appreciate food.** Acknowledge the gift of food and the effort needed to grow and prepare it. Enjoy your food with gratitude.

4. **Eat slowly.** Eating slowly may help you better recognize your hunger and satiety cues. Try to put your fork down between bites, chew your food well, and make each meal last at least 20 minutes.

5. **Be mindful about the taste, texture, and smell of food.** Savor your food. Notice the flavor, shape, and texture of each bite.

6. **Be mindful of portions to enjoy quality, not quantity.** When more food is served, we are tempted to eat more. Be mindful of the portion sizes being served on your plate.

7. **Be mindful of how hungry you are.** External cues such as seeing or smelling food may be signaling you to eat, but are you really hungry?

8. **Eat before you get too hungry.** When you get too hungry, you may be tempted to make impulsive choices instead of mindful selections.

---

[32] Dunn C, Thomas C, Aggarwal S, Nordby K, Johnson M, Myer S, Haubenreiser M. 12 Mindful Eating Strategies. 2018.

[33] Created by Eat Smart, Move More, Weigh Less, an online weight management program delivered in real-time by a Registered Dietitian Nutritionist (RDN).

9. **Be mindful of your protein**. Choose plant-based proteins often such as beans and legumes.

10. **Be mindful of your calorie budget.** Everyone has a number of calories that can be eaten each day to maintain a healthy weight. One way to be mindful of the calories you are consuming is to track what you eat and drink. Tracking for even a few days can increase your mindfulness of what and how much you are consuming.

11. **Determine if the food is calorie-worthy.** When it comes to special holiday foods or "sometimes" foods, ask yourself, is this calorie-worthy? If you are going to splurge on a high-calorie food, make sure it is something you really enjoy – then have just a few bites.

12. **Take one bite.** Follow the one-bite rule when it comes to special foods or desserts. You will not feel deprived from missing out on a favorite food and will not feel guilty for eating too much. The maximum pleasure of eating a food usually comes in the first bite.

To lose weight there should be no snacking as this slips into mindless discounted food intake. To lose weight eating must be deliberate and thought about. This may be formalized to three meals a day but in any event, be it one meal or six, eating must be thought about, deliberate, controlled and enjoyed.

Practice restraint – eat the best – think about it being the best.

In the first review of research papers on mindful eating and weight loss[34] "all studies showed weight loss results" with mindful eating. In addition, four of five studies over a follow-up period found continued weight loss. The expected regain occurred in only one of the five studies.

Mindfulness may work, the papers propose, because it strengthens the weakest link in most diets which is maintaining any weight lost. Regaining weight lost happens in part for metabolic and hormonal reasons, but mainly because few can follow restrictive eating patterns for long. Thus, any behavioral trick that helps you stick to the original plan will enhance your long-term success.

---

[34] Curr Obes Rep. 2018 Mar;7(1):37-49. doi: 10.1007/s13679-018-0299-6.
Mindfulness Approaches and Weight Loss, Weight Maintenance, and Weight Regain.

The review concluded, "Increased mindful eating has been shown to help participants gain awareness of their bodies, be more in tune to hunger and satiety, recognize external cues to eat, gain self-compassion, decrease food cravings, decrease problematic eating, and decrease reward-driven eating."

Non-Hungry Eating

Whereas Mindless Eating may unconsciously seeks 'compensation' for perceived 'exercise' or just an unthinking routine, Non-Hungry Eating is the ritualistic eating because it is if front of the person. Children know when they are full and simply don't want more (unless it is sugary drinks and junk) but adults lose this ability and, despite not being hungry, will still eat. We have been brought up 'not to waste' but leaving a third of the food on your plate is a good way to start portion control but you still have to think if you are actually hungry or even wait 20 minutes and reassess it.

The classic 'bad' habit is when we have a snack when we get home from work. This starts as an innocent occasional one-off, but then becomes a ritual and then an unconscious daily habit.

Eat More Slowly[35]

When subjects ate more slowly - changing their eating speed — fast, normal to slow — during the six-year study, those who moved from the fast to the slow category had a 42% lower rate of obesity than those who continued to eat quickly. Those who moved from fast to normal had a 29% lower rate. The researchers speculated that fast eaters consume calories more quickly than the body can register fullness, while slow eaters will notice "feelings of satiety before an excessive amount of food is ingested."

GET USED TO EATING LESS

EAT MORE SLOWLY

THINK ABOUT IT

---

[35] BMJ Open Effects of changes in eating speed on obesity in patients with diabetes: a secondary analysis of longitudinal health check-up data. Volume 8, Issue 1

CHAPTER 10

TRIGGERS

Triggers are sensations that incite you to eat and can result in you developing an eating habit.

Eating habits are invariably bad.

They can be short term, an immediate habit or 'reward', or long term, the lifestyle or stress that initiated this trigger e.g. you may have a snack and a drink when you get home as an immediate habit but is this due to long hours and stress.

Whatever, if it becomes *a habit* it causes you to eat, mostly without thinking and when you are not hungry, and some fix must be found; either less stress or do something else other than eat and drink – "DSD" - change 'time for a drink' to 'time for a walk'.

Warning

In a recent experiment exposing people to triggers, their negative emotional state, and the degree to which they experienced intrusive thoughts and tried to avoid thinking about the content were analyzed. The results across all six experiments were consistent: Trigger warnings had little effect. That is, participants responded to the content similarly, regardless of whether they saw a trigger warning.

While these were triggers to much more dramatic events the lesson here is that we can and do ignore triggers. It will now be essential for you to consciously identify but then diligently avoid or obviate them. The danger is recognizing them but being immune or blaze and ignoring these danger signals.

Advertising
- Ads urge us to eat more than we need
- >90% of children's TV Ads were for food
- Streets of Fast Food outlets and drive-ins encourage drop-ins
- If it has to be advertised it's processed junk
- People were more likely to pick unhealthful or calorie-laden items when the ambient music was loud, and healthful items when softer music was played[36]

---

[36] Journal of the Academy of Marketing Science January 2019, Volume 47, Issue 1, pp 37–55| Cite as Sounds like a healthy retail atmospheric strategy: Effects of ambient music and background noise on food sales

Avoidance

- Avoid triggers:
    - In the short-term DSD Do Something Different
    - In the long-term work out why something triggers you and alter your lifestyle
- Confront problems or compulsions like eating when stressed, drinking to relax and plan substitutions / avoidance
- Make a list of everything that triggers or stimulates you to eat. Hang it up in the kitchen. Read it before you pig out.
- Have alternate list of Things to Do and do them instead
- List foods you find irresistible or comforting and avoid. Regard them as your enemies and make special efforts to avoid them
- Avoid the 'comfort foods' you liked as a kid
- When people encounter stimuli that they have learned to associate with certain snacks, they tend to choose those products, even when they know these are unhealthy
- Some people can't stop if they start. Don't start! If you don't take the first bite you won't have a problem
- Paradoxically these people often find fasting their preferred regime
- Don't graze. Don't go to the fridge and look
- Irresistible snacks are always placed at eye height! Move them!
- Substitutes: Soda water and fresh lime juice instead of booze
- Realize you are not out of control with all foods. Just identify, isolate and make special plans for them
- Binge Eating is a secret problem. You will only avoid them if you identify what triggers them and have avoidance plans or substitutions
- Paste inspirational messages of the fridge: 'Not Now!', 'Are You Really Hungry?', 'Go Walk'
- Never leave those irresistible leftovers in the fridge
- Change routines not to pass shops / temptations
- Regard Trigger Foods now as your enemy. They initiate fat gain
- There is no such thing as 'Just One'
- Identify, control, limit or discard all junk triggers

THE IRRESISTIBLE, FAT-GAINING SNACKS ARE ALWAYS AT EYE-HEIGHT ON THE REFRIGERATOR SHELVES

MOVE THEM: DON'T BUY AS MUCH

Situation Specific triggers
- TV, weekends, parties, stress, boredom, loneliness, anger, frustration, tiredness, coming home, aromas, cooking

Assertion
- Learn to say 'No'
- Don't say you are dieting, it leads to sabotage
- Have excuses ready. Be firm, polite and offer alternatives: "The meal was wonderful, but I'd love some coffee/tea/fruit"
- Always leave some food on your plate (excuse: "I had a massive lunch")
- Learn to cook not to reheat processed junk meals. Steak and salads.
- Plan and, if possible, prepare meals a week ahead

Shopping
- Shopping is where weight loss begins. Shop thin
- If you don't buy it, you can't eat it
- Make a list and stick to it
- Don't use a shopping trolley
- Never shop when you are hungry
- Supermarket: No kids, don't cruise, fresh food aisles only

Substitution
- Best substitutes to eating are exercise or occupation
- Not deprived but emancipated: Good food for junk
- Substitute fruit for junk
- Get rid of all junk foods
- No late-night munching, which can sabotage your calorie intake

- Read labels. Breakfast cereals, ketchup are full of sugar
- Reduce intake by only 300 – 500 calories a day. This maximizes weight loss and minimizes side-effects
- Don't eat from containers: Measure out portions
- Smaller plates, smaller glasses, smaller portions
- Share desserts

Support
- You need support in your own home to lose weight.
- Get someone to check your intake (don't hide anything).
- Get a monitor/motivator. Your doctor, nutritionist if needed
- It would be preferable if your house-mate joined in
- Having help estimating calories and planning and preparing meals

---

THE KEY IS TO NOW IDENTIFY TRIGGERS

and

SUBSTITUTE NON-EATING HABITS

by

DOING SOMETHING DIFFERENT - DSD

HUMANS HAVE BEEN PROGRAMMED

FOR MILLIONS OF YEARS

TO STORE UP FAT FOR WINTER

BUT NOW

WINTER NEVER COMES

CHAPTER 11

EATING RULES

Slow Down at the table
It takes a minimum of 20 minutes for the brain to pick up on satiety, the fullness of the stomach, and you miss the cue of being full if you're eating too quickly even if it is healthy-but-rich foods.

Eat More Slowly[37]
Up to a 42% lower rate of obesity compared with those who tended to eat quickly or gobble up their food. Those who ate at a normal speed were 29 percent less likely to be obese, rising to 42 percent for those who ate slowly (something to chew on?). Snacking after dinner and eating within 2 hours of going to sleep 3 or more times a week were also strongly linked to changes in BMI. But skipping breakfast wasn't.

> **A 42% LOWER RATE OF OBESITY WHEN EATING REDUCED FROM FAST TO SLOW**

Plan Ahead: "Essential".
Most people only have a vague idea of what they are going to eat the next day and any good intentions are soon detoured and destroyed by the innumerable food temptations, stresses and changes to that day.

One of the most successful control mechanisms is to plan your meals ahead by at least a day, or more if you can. And then stick to it!

This allows you time to strictly measure the calories in your next day meals and enforces that you don't succumb to temptation or "forget" to register that snack or only make estimates of calories on the fly.

Planning Ahead is extremely effective and may well be essential, especially when you embark on a new regime.

---

[37] BMJ Open Effects of changes in eating speed on obesity in patients with diabetes: a secondary analysis of longitudinal health check-up data. Volume 8, Issue 1

Self-Monitoring:

Log Often, Lose More: Smartphone Apps Weight Loss[38]

A recent study confirmed that the frequency of self-monitoring was significantly related to weight-loss success with both the number of days per month and the number of times per day of recording on the smartphone app. Those losing ≥ 10% of their baseline weight were journaling approximately three times a day. The time needed to log in and record was only 15 minutes later in the program. This study mentioned the Apps Lose It, Calorie King, and My Fitness Pal. I used Calorie King which took a day or so frustration but then it was good. Calorie King has two Apps. Don't use the Nutrition Program – use the Kalorie Count App.

Warning: To be most effective (which is what you want) you _must_ record it before or as you eat it. Or…

DID I EAT THAT

DIET

WRITE WHEN YOU BITE

LOG OFTEN, LOSE MORE

---

better still – Plan Ahead.

Stomach Shrinkage: Six Weeks to Adapt

Our empty stomachs are the size of a large apple but can stretch to some two liters – the size of two large soft drink-soda bottles.

Our stomachs obviously can, and actually do, stretch more than this if we progressively over-eat. Which most of us do today due to the abundance of food. The walls of our stomach have 'pressor receptors' or, in other words, pressure receptors that, when the walls of the stomach stretch, signals to the brain that it is full.

---

[38] Obesity: Log Often, Lose More: Electronic Dietary Self-Monitoring for Weight Loss published: 25 February 2019

By chronically overeating the stomach stretches and we need more food to impress them to signal the brain.

In the same way, if we eat less, our stomachs will shrink, and we won't feel we have to eat the same quantity to feel full.

Unfortunately, this takes some time...at least six weeks and in the interim the brain is sending back messages for our stomach and intestines to produce more ghrelin, the hormone that makes us hungry and makes us want to eat.

Stick with it. Eventually your stomach will shrink and expect smaller volumes without triggering the pressor receptors and ghrelin. This is the long-term goal to aim for: Eating less satisfies you.

YUM YUM

EXPANDS MY TUM

You Will Fall Off the Wagon

We all fall off the wagon. So what? Nobody's perfect. It is not this fall from grace or our pig-out that's the problem, it's how this should determine you to re-confirm your commitment and to concentrate on getting back to your plan.

Take time out and reassess if you can keep to the diet you selected. If not try another. You may go from 5:2, to 16:8 to 600cals less a day or even one day complete fast.

And you may want to mix them up.

DON'T GIVE UP, GET BACK UP

CHAPTER 12

SIDE EFFECTS and DIFFICULTIES

Hunger

The most immediate and most common side-effect from reducing your intake is the increase in hunger. Acute energy deficits imposed by food restriction increases your appetite and food intake.

Exercise does not induce hunger and is the best "cure".

But Is It Hunger

If you have reduced your intake these are often withdrawal-symptoms, as for any drug of addiction, but these hunger pains and cravings are from your addiction / overuse of food. Like any drug of addiction, you must recognize and fight these and not give in and have some more food "just this once". Hunger means you are succeeding! You may liken it to having sore muscles after running or exercising.

Hormones that are released to stimulate you to eat after a meal persist for as long as 12 months after weight loss. [39] The main appetite stimulant is Ghrelin. A hormone that is produced and released mainly by the stomach with small amounts also released by the small intestine, pancreas and brain. Ghrelin has numerous functions. It is termed the 'hunger hormone' because it stimulates appetite, increases food intake and promo

What we feel is 'hunger' is often some other mood disturbance such as boredom and thinking about food when, if you were out having a great time or working, you wouldn't feel "hungry". So rather than actual hunger this is a manufactured habit-response to your boredom or other mood disturbance. Smokers lose weight because 'oral gratification' which starts when we are babies on the nipple, is a response to stress or other mood disturbances. If you've not eaten for 16 hours (the 16:8 regime, you may feel hungry but it is hard to conceive that snacking between breakfast and lunch or afternoon tea are due to real hunger.

---

[39] NEJM, 2011, 365:1597-1604

DIFFICULTIES
Set Point
Our body seems to recognize a weight where it feels we want to be. Both when we are putting on weight ("I can't believe I didn't put on any weight" we often say) but then also on the way back down. These are called "Set Points or Default Values"

Set point theory says that there is a control system in each individual that regulates our body weight – like a 'body thermostat for body fat'. According to the theory, when we lose weight, if our Set Point is the new body weight, our new weight can remain constant. Our bodies have an appropriate amount of energy storage relative to the amount of activity we do and the amount of calories we consume. If our Set Point at the new weight remains high, however, our bodies will gradually bring us back to a higher weight, maybe even back to our original weight.

Plateauing
Sticking at a set point is known as Plateauing.

To survive, the human is genetically programmed to lay down fat against famine and hard times. This also resists any attempts to lose it.

If you are to succeed losing fat you will have to persist in a series of step-like stages as 'default' or "set-point" weights are reached. Default weights are those you attained as you gained weight and the brain recognized these as the weight *you* wanted to be and set this level. You probably can't remember but your body actually resisted gaining weight then, but not as much as now.

But is also resists you trying to lose weight. Now, on the way down, it again recognizes this default value and again resists changes.

So, despite you continuing to eat less, you don't lose. You plateau.

Solution: To lose more weight, either increase your exercise or decrease the calories you eat. Using the same approach that worked initially may maintain your weight loss, but it won't lead to more weight loss.

There is not any conclusive evidence as to how to resume weight loss. What works for one person often doesn't work for another but sustained increases in physical activity will gradually lower the set point. You now have to increase your exercise than previously. This persistence signals the brain you are determined to reset your default value – and then you will drop again, plateau, drop, plateau, drop and so on until you reach your objective desired weight.

Our slower metabolism from eating less slows our weight loss, even if you eat the same number of calories that helped you lose weight. When the calories you burn equal the calories you eat, you reach a plateau.

1. **Reassess your habits.** Look back at your food and activity records. Make sure you haven't loosened the rules, letting yourself get by with larger portions or less exercise. Research suggests that off-and-on loosening of rules contributes to plateaus.

2. **Cut more calories.** Further cut your daily calories, provided this doesn't put you below 1,200 calories. Fewer than 1,200 calories a day may not be enough to keep you from constant hunger, which increases your risk of overeating, unless you can cope with the 800 Diet. However, lowering your calories to reduce the set point or break the plateau doesn't seem to be effective because it often reduces the body's muscle mass. If set point is lowered by these methods, people may become depressed, lethargic and suffer greater periods of hunger.

3. **Rev up your workout.** Exercise: it builds muscle and revs up your metabolism. Most people should exercise 30 minutes a day, nearly every day of the week. But people trying to lose weight should exercise more often than that or increase the intensity of exercise to burn more calories. Adding exercises such as weightlifting to increase your muscle mass will help you burn more calories.

4. **Start strength training** a few times a week. ...

5. **Pack more activity into your day.** Think outside the gym. Increase your general physical activity throughout the day by walking more and using your car less or try doing more yard work or vigorous spring cleaning. Any physical activity will help you burn more calories. Try tracking activity to see if your total minutes or steps can be increased. Find activities that have longer duration, or higher intensity. Expand your list of activities and amount, because that elevates the amount of metabolic activity throughout the day.

6. **Check your portion sizes**

7. **Make a diary / phone app of every calorie you eat**

8. **Weigh yourself daily**

Hormones

These default values are controlled by the hormones Leptin and Ghrelin.

Leptin is produced in our fat cells. When levels fall it signals the brain to eat.

Ghrelin, is produced in our stomach and intestines. When we don't eat levels rise and signals the brain for us to eat.

Slowed Metabolism from Dieting

The problem is that ghrelin production increases as weight is lost *making us want to eat, but as well, it slows our metabolism,* making it progressively harder to lose weight.

Hence these default plateaus.

Hitting the Wall

After six weeks of dieting or when a 10% weight loss is reached the body hits its resistance default value and tries to regain the lost weight or fat; the BMR Basal or Resting Metabolic Rate reduces, and people feel lethargic. They have 'hit the wall'. Low fat diets seem the worst at provoking this default-reset. But then cortisol (the stress hormone) levels rise and thyroid hormone (which elevates the BMR) levels fall. Forewarned is forearmed. You will wonder what in goodness name has happened as you slip into a soporific lethargy. Keep going. Reset the default value. You have to work through.

When weight is lost metabolism can slow which can oppose, counter and even reverse any weight loss. The BMR – Basal or Resting Metabolic Rate slows in all dieters if they exercise or not which is why weight loss may seem easy to begin with but becomes increasingly harder. Our Metabolic Rate reduces as we lose weight as we then burn less calories than when heavier. This can make you feel as if you have been slammed into a wall – hence "Hitting the Wall". The solution is the same as for Plateauing.

Disillusionment

Disillusionment is arguably the most undermining and destructive to all efforts to lose weight. Most arises from our impatience and frustration at not seeming to be losing weight – certainly at the rate at which we would like to. Plateauing and Hitting the Wall certainly make this worse.

This is why I have counseled not to embark on this unless you treat it as you would starting to run in the hope of running a marathon.

In other words, planning, being prepared and prevention are the key. You must expect that there will be periods of differing durations when you will wonder if 'it's all worth-while'.

- Go back and read the reasons you wanted to lose weight.
- Go back and see if you have lost any weight and regard *any* loss as a victory.
- One small step at a time.
- Don't wallow in self-pity. Reassess, re-assemble and reform your attack on your weight. Try harder. Eat fewer calories – exercise more.

Biggest Losers Regain Weight - The Body Wants to Return to Its Original Weight

Most, if not all of the 16 contestants in 2009 have regained most if not more weight. This was because their resting metabolism slowed as they lost weight but then never recovered. The winner, Danny Cahill, who lost 239 pounds in seven months now burns less than 800 calories a day than expected, anything else turns to fat, and has regained 100 pounds. They reported constantly battling hunger, cravings and binges. There is an argument that these people need on-going support but that there is still a need for more research.

Biggest Losers Regain Weight[40]

The Body Wants to Return to Its Original Weight

Most of the 16 contestants in 2009 regained most if not more weight. This was because their resting metabolism slowed as they lost weight but then never recovered.

The ones who maintained their weight loss increased their exercise by 160% whereas those who regained only increased it by some 35%.

The mean loss was some 58+or-25kg. After 6 years the mean regain was some 41 + or – 31kg. This infers that even among the most highly motivated long-term maintenance is extremely difficult

To compensate for your reduced BMR you now have to increase your exercise and persist to signal the brain you are determined to reset your default value – and then you will drop again, plateau, drop, plateau, drop and so on until you reach your objective desired weight.

[40] Obesity (Silver Spring), 2016; 24:1612-1619

Solution

Re-read this chapter if and when these side-effects hit. Understand what's going on: Know your enemy and fight back.

Hunger, Cravings and Binges

The Biggest Losers reported constantly battling hunger, cravings and binges. They, of course, have profound metabolic medical problems beyond the parameters of this book which, as stated at the outset, is for those of us with a BMI around 30, who were once slimmer and have insidiously put on weight, but you too will have to battle hunger, cravings and will have to try to minimize binges.

Knowing this will help. The hunger, the cravings and the binge breakouts are all part of it.

What you have to do is

- only eat a very little to abate the hunger
- give into your craving but, again, minimize it
- try to also minimize a binge but then don't give up, go away, readjust, reorganize and get back up

---

IF YOU ARE HUNGRY YOU ARE EATING LESS
AND LOSING WEIGHT!

RECOGNIZE HUNGER AS 'YOUR FRIEND'
PART OF THE 'CURE'

BUT YOU WILL SOON ADJUST AND NOT FEEL HUNGRY AND...
IT'S ONLY FOR TODAY

CHAPTER 13

STAY MOTIVATED

REAL REASONS why diets fail
- Lack of resolve
- Lack of discipline
- Impatience

Most Listed Excuses to stop Losing Weight
- Lack of time
- Program dissatisfaction

Most usual reactions for excuses
- Not fast enough
- Denial
- Anger
- Rebellion
- Disillusionment
- Burn-out
- Revenge
- Relapse

HOW TO KEEP DIETING
- Weigh every day
- Some "advisors" recommend you don't weigh every day. I think this is as absurd as if an athlete or swimmer wouldn't record their training times
- Put up a Graph
- You will have to make time. Get focused
- Allocate absolutely uninterrupted time each day and week to refine your program and reinforce your efforts
- Dedicate some "Me Time" to recuperate and reorganize
- Most failures are due to lack of willpower and determination
- Next is becoming disappointed or disillusioned at either not losing fast enough or "plateauing" - not losing despite dieting
- Overweight people frequently know more about and are obsessed by food but they just lack will power and persistence

- Never give up. Never give up. Never give up
- Most people who lapse don't or won't change habits
- Be happy with any loss no matter how small
- Do not make goals too hard: Set small initial short-term goals. Don't think "I've only lost a little" but rather "I am losing and heading toward my goal"
- Have small short-term goals rather than one final big one
- Losing weight is slow. It is a marathon
- The more overweight the more unrealistic the expectations
- Discard all preconceptions. This is you. ANY loss is a victory. "Every long journey starts with one small step"
- You will need constant motivation and help. Find a diet partner
- One day at a time. Just today eat less today
- Never feel full. Leave some food on your plate. (Don't worry you won't die - in fact you will live longer)
- Just 100 calories less a day loses weight
- Gain control
- Resolve. Resolve. Resolve. Never give up
- Diets are stressful. You have to keep at it until it becomes your new habit, your new foods your new satiety level (the amount of food that satisfies). This takes at least six weeks
- Find the personal key that best motivates you
  - A photo when you were slimmer
  - A photo of someone you resemble or admire and is lean
  - But no negative photos or measurements that frustrate
  - A graph of your weight, wall planner, waist size
- NEWTRITION Foods are based on the Mediterranean diet but updated and evidenced to be the healthiest of all and to lose weight. If you stick to these foods and eat less, you will lose weight

Do Not Blame Yourself

If you can't stick to the diet – change! Find one that suits. It's the diet that fails – not you.

Don't focus on restriction but better nutrition – no processed junk.

Eat more slowly and think about your meal.

Get a more than 7 hours sleep.

Sugar, Sweets and Soda-Soft Drinks

Are today's villains. But a little is OK. Just try and slowly cut down e.g. Two teaspoons of sugar in your tea gradually reduce so you don't detect the difference. But simply no colas or such.

EAT THAT

and

GET FAT

Don't Get Bored

Don't give up your favorite foods totally. Try gradually substituting different high nutrition foods even if initially you don't like them but don't force yourself. It takes around some seven 'challenges' to get to accept new foods.

Don't Be Impatient

Weight loss goes in fits and starts with plateauing. Hang in there.

MAINTENANCE MONITORING

Now learn to control your appetite which, with our modern lifestyle, affluence and excess of junk food, is very difficult.

1. Think "Restraint"
2. Think are you actually hungry or just bored, grazing and 'rewarding'
3. Are meals smaller
4. Are there fewer snacks and more formal meals
5. Are there less fat and refined carbohydrates
6. Is exercise > 30 mins a day or better still do SIT
7. Look up daily Calorie needs for age, height and sex and don't exceed – in fact eat 600 cals less.
8. Although weight loss is achievable for many adults, weight maintenance is elusive
9. After completing weight loss programs about a third of the weight lost is regained in the following year but an 81% success rate is possible

Again, as weight falls metabolism slows
Appetite changes – need 100 cals more for every 1kg drop
People react differently to same food eg Blood Glucose (BG) response
10% wt drop = BP and BG improvement

Photo Therapy
I well remember a colleague's wife, when I was specializing in Edinburgh, who had a photo of Jacki Kennedy on her kitchen wall and indeed she progressively looked like Jacki! While she bore a distinct resemblance to Jacki it was Jacki's photo of this slim elegant woman that kept inspiring my friend to emulate her.

If you have a photo of someone you feel you could get to look like if you lost weight, or someone with a flat tummy or a six-pack or even a photo of yourself if you were slim, then put it up in the kitchen and look at it before you eat!

THINK

I CAN HAVE IT

BUT I DON'T WANT IT

CHAPTER 14

TRAPS

Entitlement Justification
*   Eating more because you exercise: Dieters ate 79g when they knew they were going to exercise cf 28g when they did not expect to run.
*   Too sudden a change with too many changes
*   Changing to a diet that you can't stick to forever (? Keto)
*   Trying multiple fad diets
*   Not increasing physical activity
*   Alcohol is an appetite stimulant very high in Empty Calories

Rewards – Comfort
Everybody has their "comfort foods" which we seek when we are stressed, tired, exhausted and such. They donate us a "reward" for all the incredible hard work and problems we have had to grapple with…and make us fat.
No! It's not much of a reward if it makes you fat.

DSD! Do Something Different!

Cravings
Several behavioral studies have demonstrated that denying certain foods, like being on a diet, causes increased craving and motivation for that food. Craving for foods high in fat - this includes many junk foods - is an important part of obesity and binge eating. When trying to lose weight people often strive to avoid fatty foods, which ironically increases motivation and craving for these foods and can lead to overeating. Even worse, the longer someone abstains from fatty foods, the greater the cravings.

As in Chapter 12 with hunger and binges, forewarned is forearmed: If you know this is going to happen you can indulge in this naughty treat but try and control and limit it and earn it.

"Go with the flow". Don't ban your cravings all together – you'll only miss them more and they can become an obsession and you then pig out. Have some but try and minimize.

Stability

Young adults who maintained stable BMI over time had minimal progression of risk factors and lower incidence of metabolic syndrome regardless of BMI baseline. Long term weight stabilization should be the aim.

Less Sleep

It seems that disrupted sleep contributes to excessive food intake. Seven to eight hours would seem optimum. Try and get this.

Food Porn

Food is not meant to be looked at but ingested, experienced and enjoyed.
Highly stylized, air brushed, glamorized, glorified images or 'food porn' trigger the 'hunger hormone' ghrelin that increases appetite and stimulates gastric acid secretion. It reaches higher levels in the bloodstream of people shown images of food compared with non-food images and drives increased food intake and reduces the body's utilization of fat stores.

To counteract the effects of these highly manipulated and seductive images of food, avoid sleep deprivation, keep physically active and be aware of hunger and fullness signals.

Cooking was another protective activity. The more food is handled food the less people are affected or 'desensitized' by food porn and the less they actually need to eat to get satisfaction.

That Said

I have noted how the Celebrity Chefs have slowly put on weight, except for Gordon Ramsay. I wondered how, until he revealed in one program how he runs four marathons a year! While exercise may only be 15% of weight loss – marathons are something else – I have never seen a fat marathoner.

Sex

Eating is the second most powerful urge on earth (the biological urge to procreate is stronger even than the urge to survive or eat). I do not bring this up salaciously, but to point how losing weight is arguably the hardest thing to do in this era of affluence and availability of addictive, junk food available, home-delivered, 24 hours a day, 7 days a week along with the labor saving devices, cars, remote controls, computers and sedentary lifestyles and where the Fast Food Industry spends $trillions to seduce you down the Supermarket central aisles to eat processed food often labeled 'healthy' and which tastes delicious and is researched to make you want more.

No one else can provide you with the willpower. However, 'Information is power' which may give you an understanding of the problem and this phenomenon and provide you with the facts and not the dreams and scams of the fad diets that will lead you up the garden path…to the fat farm.

Weigh Daily

The more frequently dieters weighed themselves the more weight they lost, and if participants went more than a week without weighing themselves, they gained weight

---

IF IT HAS TO BE LABELED "HEALTHY"

IT AIN'T HEALTHY

Healthy Foods

You can over eat these too.

Exercise

Does not mean you can eat more

Alcohol

Booze is just 'empty calories' what is worse it is an appetite stimulant. Learn to control it and record it!

YOU WON'T LOSE

WHEN YOU DRINK BOOZE

"Everyday in every way I'm getting better and better".

– Emile Coue

Around a century ago a French psychologist, Emile Coue, believed that most mental and physical illness was a result of the person's thinking and he discovered that he could help the recovery of a patient simply by praising the effectiveness of the treatment to the patient.

He understood how we are often our own worst enemy. How, if we think negative thoughts over time these negative thoughts take their toll. He found that Autosuggestion, or affirmations would counteract this negativity and he coined the phrase that could be most helpful.

Losing weight is incredibly difficult and frustrating and we can't help getting depressed and feeling negative thoughts. Autosuggestion via this positive affirmation actually works elsewhere so why not for weight loss. It will concentrate and positively focus your intent rather than feeling sad and wallowing in self-pity.

Advocates point out that if you mumble this phrase to yourself half-heartedly a few times it's pretty obvious it will do nothing for you. But if you concentrate on *really* meaning it. If you focus completely on the affirmation and say it with real feeling and conviction for 10 minutes then you will start to notice an effect. They recommend the best approach is to do this for 10 minutes every evening before you go to bed. If you do this for two weeks then they claim you'll be raving about how awesome it is.

LOSING WEIGHT IS A CONSTANT DISCIPLINE

BUT

'EVERY DAY, IN EVERY WAY, I WILL LOSE WEIGHT'

CHAPTER 15

MAINTENANCE OF WEIGHT LOSS

Post-bariatric surgery behaviors, which would also seem relevant to anyone trying to lose weight, that were significantly linked to weight regain included
- sedentary time
- frequently eating fast food
- eating when full
- eating continuously
- disordered eating such as binge and loss of control eating

Weighing oneself at least once weekly was linked to significantly less weight regain.

Exercise and physical activity, even if just house work or gardening, are especially important.

The latest research has found that Metformin helped maintain long-term weight loss in individuals at risk for type 2 diabetes.

IF YOU ARE UPSET

DON'T EAT

E.

NUTRITION

CHAPTER 16

NEWTRITION

I TOLD YOU SO

Since the first (sold out) edition of my book "Newtrition" it is gratifying, but not surprising, to find my recommendations now confirmed in five subsequent large surveys published in the world's best medical journals.

All these recommendations are covered if you eat these Super-Mediterranean Foods.

And while these studies have more to do with good health or, rather how the eating of junk foods promotes an early death, they also confirm my advice that vitamins and supplements are of benefit but only if obtained from our (Super-Mediterranean) food. Vitamin pill and supplements are of no use, and may even be harmful

As to obesity, my hypothesis is that we humans have taken some 2(+) million years of evolution, in which time we have worked out or very slowly adapted to the foods we can, or cannot, eat but the development of fast foods "Ready-to-Eat" or "Heat-and-Eat" after World War 2 introduced ultra-processed foods, chemical and additives which, I maintain, we can't metabolize and which, due to its cheapness, availability and deliciousness, we over-eat as well.

The current epidemic of obesity almost perfectly shadows and tracks this introduction of processed fast / junk foods.

To lose weight it will be necessary to not eat any junk / processed foods, to eat the Newtrition Super-Mediterranean foods across all groups and, to eat less.

But Further: The latest research from Harvard would seem to support my Obesity Hypothesis: They found that a common preservative used to prevent bread and cakes going mouldy could be fuelling the obesity crisis by harming metabolisms, scientists at Harvard University have warned.[41] Propionate is widely used in baked goods, animal feed and artificial flavouring – but research indicates that it leads to increased levels of hormones that trigger weight gain and diabetes. Researchers at Harvard TH Chan School of Public Health carried out two studies,

---

[41] Science Translational Medicine, April 2019.

one in animals and one in humans, which showed propionate triggers a "cascade of metabolic events" that can lead to insulin resistance and weight gain. A further study in 14 humans found those who consumed the meal containing propionate had significant increases in norepinephrine as well as increases in glucagon and gluconeogenic soon after eating the meal.

This is just one of some potential 85,000 new chemicals introduced into processed foods since WW2. And while certainly not all 85,000 are in our processed foods, who knows? Some may have no effect, some may even be beneficial (I doubt it) but many of these "additives" are new, synthetic chemicals which, I think, our bodies simply can't metabolise.

To put it simply, "Fresh is Best".

And now more additives are becoming under suspicion elsewhere: PARIS (Reuters 20/4/2019) - France will ban the use of titanium dioxide as a food additive from 2020 after the country's health and safety agency said there was not enough evidence to guarantee the safety of the substance. Titanium dioxide is widely used in industry as a whitener, notably for paint, and in the food sector, where it is labelled E171 and goes into products from chocolate to chewing gum. France's National Institute for Agricultural Research (INRA) and partners in a study of oral exposure to titanium dioxide had shown that E171 crosses the intestine wall in animals to reach other parts of the body and after a 2017 study found health effects in animals that consumed it.

I am not saying, of course, that processed foods are the only cause of our obesity epidemic: But these Fast Foods are available 24 hours a day, home delivered, incredibly affordable, taste delicious and are so convenient that we are also over-eating far more than previous generations. I do maintain, however, that processed foods are an overlooked contributor. Nothing else has changed.

THE SUPER-MEDITERRANEAN FOODS

These NEWTRITION-Super-Mediterranean Foods, listed below, are evidenced to be the most beneficial for our health. They provide "small, pleasant, acceptable substitutions" for weight-gaining or damaging foods. If you have favorite but damaging foods, such as SSB - Sugar Sweetened Beverages (Sodas and Soft Drink), sausages and preserved meats, deep fried foods and so on, as part of losing weight you *must* find health substitutions.

If you are addicted to junk food, you will have to make an effort to reduce then cease it while learning to discover or re-discover the delights of natural fruit and produce. There is nothing more delicious than a ripe mango then nectarine, tangelo and such. Nuts make good snacks. But you will have to make the effort. Processed food is poison.

THE NEWTRITION SUPER-MEDITERRANEAN FOODS

20% Fruit
20% Vegetables
20% Grains, Seeds and Nuts
20% Protein - mostly plants
20% Superfoods (Micronutrients)

THE NEWTRITION SUPERFOODS:

These foods have been identified as being richer in micronutrients and which donate greater benefits than others.

The Newtrition Superfoods are:

Apples/pears (white fruit), Apricots (dried), Beetroot, Berries*, Celery, Chilies, Chocolate-dark/cocoa, Citrus, Coffee, Fiber, Fish, Garlic/onion family, Grains, Green Leafy Vegetables-Bok Choy, Inulin vegetables (chicory, leeks, asparagus, Jerusalem artichokes), Legumes, Mushrooms, Nuts (walnuts, pecans, peanuts), Oats (barley) (rolled/cut), Olive Oil, Peppers/Capsicums Orange (Men), Prunes, Sweet Potato (purple), Vegetables green-yellow-cruciferous)

Maybe: Magnesium, Curcumin, Cinnamon, Pomegranate Juice with Dates, Rosemary, Sage, Vinegar, Chamomile, Peppermint and Kombucha teas, Kifir (fermented milk)

EVERY DAY ESSENTIALS:

YES

- Fruit variety, ensure berries, apples (skin), citrus
- Veg: esp green leafy, purple sweet potato, orange peppers, legumes, lentils
- Nuts. 20g. walnuts, pecans, peanuts, almonds
- Grains
- Chilies
- Cocoa, Chocolate (dark)
- Coffee
- Extra Virgin Olive Oil (EVOO)
- Fish
- Fiber
- Superfoods
- Mushrooms twice a week

Leave something on your plate: Never get full

Calm, pleasant meals. Happy people only.

NO

- Processed foods or meats
- Butter, cream
- Added sugar
- Sugar Sweetened Beverages (SSB)
- Added salt

VITAMIN PILLS AND SUPPLEMENTS ARE A SCAM

(Unless you have a _proven_ deficiency)

Do not trust the "Health" shop. Do not listen to any advice other than a qualified medical practitioner and even then, I'd be cautious if he or she was "alternate"

EAT THE NEWTRITION SUPER-MEDITERRANEAN FOODS

They provide ALL nutritional needs AND donate health benefits

---

Golden Rules

- Ensure great variety of freshest, local, ripest produce
- Benefits exceed any residual pesticides but wash
- Pleasant, calm environment; enjoy your food, company
- No eating in cars. No Gas Station foods
- Don't eat until you feel full. Leave some food
- "It's not what you cut out, it's what you replace it with".
- Do not replace fat with refined carbohydrates
- Avoid all processed foods. Anything in a package is processed.
- All processing is bad until proven otherwise
- No smoked, preserved meats (bacon, ham, sausages) and processed cheese
- Think more vegetarian
- Vegetables every day esp. dark green leafy "cabbage"
- All fruit and vegetables are good, full of antioxidants
- Variety of fruit every day. Eat whole fruit, not just juice
- The skin contains over 90% of the nutrients
- Orange capsicums / peppers reduce Ca prostate
- Berries x 3 times a week (slows cognitive decline)
- An apple a day can reduce all-cause mortality, heart attacks and strokes. Oranges, pears too
- Reduce potatoes (associated with hypertension)
- Purple Sweet Potato / purple vegetables good
- 15 g nuts daily. Stroke & prostate cancer risk reduced. Walnuts, pecans best(?).
- Grains 70g/day lowers risk all-cause death, cancer, CVD
- High-fiber reduces heart attacks, colorectal Ca (CAC)
- Olive oil 20 ml / day. Reduced risk of stroke and CAD
- Polyunsaturated oils the best for heart protection
- No butter, no cream. Fermented dairy OK
- Skim or "heart healthy" milk
- Milk 200g, 50g cheese or 400 g dairy reduces risk of CAC (Ca Colon)
- Every 300 mg Calcium (to 1900mg) from food, reduces risk CAC.
- No supplements: getting too much calcium from supplements (at least 1,000 milligrams a day) increases your risk of dying of cancer. But that relationship doesn't exist if you're getting that much calcium from food
- If you take vitamin D without being vitamin D deficient, you could be increasing your chances of dying of cancer. More research is needed.

- Eat more fish: X 2 a week. Avoid Fish Oil capsules.
- Less red meat. All-cause mortality, Ca and CVD higher for meat eaters
- Eat only organic poultry and eggs
- More vinegar. Maybe a secret of the Mediterranean Diet
- More fresh herbs, garlic
- Chilies lower risk of total mortality and Ca risk
- Breakfast cereals of oats best. Avoid commercial processed brands.
- Breakfast is not necessary
- A glass of red wine with food daily.
- Women with family history of breast Ca, men who smoke, should abstain
- Coffee 4 cups a day. Green or no-milk tea
- Vitamin D 1000 IU /day. Some recommend 4000 IU/day
- Dark chocolate or 2 heap teaspoons cocoa, daily
- Salt: Current guidelines are for 2.3g / day. Check labels
- Taste before you add salt; break the "autopilot" habit
- Increase potassium: fruits (dried apricots)
- Reduce sugar intake < 4 g sugar per 100 g in any serving
- Avoid HFCS (High Fructose Corn Syrup in many drinks)
- Micro-filtered water (to avoid *Giardia* & *Cryptosporidium*).
- Don't shop hungry. No portion distortion, small, no 2nds
- Dry bake vegetables or microwave.
- Avoid soya bean oil may increase obesity and diabetes.
- Microwaving veg best preserves vitamins and minerals
- Avoid the middle aisles in supermarkets.
- No very hot beverages (carcinogenic)
- Intermittent Fasting Diets for health and weight loss
- Pomegranate juice + 3 dates or just pomegranate juice
- Mushrooms are associated with reduced cognitive impairment

WORLD'S BEST BREAKFAST
- Blueberries - for brain health
- Granny Smith (skin) - gut health and stroke prevention
- Walnuts, pecans - anti cancer, heart health.
- Oats or Bran - lowers cholesterol, better microbiome
- Grains - reduce All-Cause-Mortality, CVD and cancer
- Flax (ground) - richest source Omega-3 ALA
- Inulin - reduces visceral fat

- Dried apricots. High potassium - lowers BP
- Green bananas: Fiber speeds gut transit. Potassium
- Biodynamic unsweetened yogurt (< 4g sugar / 100g)
- Fruit in season
- Prunes - fiber / microbiome gut health
- Coffee - Super-food

WORLD'S WORST BREAKFAST FOODS

- Cereals high in sugar and salt
- Sausages
- Bacon/ham
- Eggs
- Hash browns
- Butter
- Crumpets
- Waffles / Pancakes
- Golden / Maple Syrup
- Muffins
- Sugar in your tea or coffee

Be wary of 'health' foods: 'Health' smoothies can contain over 500cals!

Be super-suspicious of all those delicious commercial sauces on hamburgers, salads and such. Remember, even just strawberry flavoring contains 59 chemicals. Many are untested, and we simply don't know what they do.

Do not worry about the occasional lapse or treat.

Successful weight loss focuses on adding healthy foods whereas the less successful over-compensate and deprive themselves.

There should be no sense of deprivation or sacrifice. Initially if you are a chocoholic you may find it difficult to replace milk chocolate. If you are drinking colas or "sports" drinks finding a substitute may also be a problem. But persist: Your tastes will change - for the better. Dark Chocolate is an acquired taste but it's beneficial. Coffee or tea are the best substitutes for Sugar-Sodas; nuts instead of crisps and fruit for lunch. The "World's Best Breakfast" - gets you breakfasters away from the sugar-saturated breakfast cereals.
Small, acceptable, pleasant substitutions.

Food Choices

If you are not prepared, or cannot, stop eating junk food then you may as well not try at all but just accept your diabetes, blood pressure, heart problems, joint problems, increased cancer risk and, of course, depression – but hey! There's a pill for most of those. But not for fat.

The $Trillion Fast Food Industry is geared to actively counter and nobble any moves that may impact on their profits. They have infiltrated (by subsidies) the most august Medical Establishments and Dietitian Associations as well as Governments by threatening closure of factories and hence unemployment, which has seen off and suppressed medical studies as to the damaging effects of their 'products'.

It is most important that you now eat only a mostly plant-based diet and avoid all processed foods.

NO SALTED NUTS

SALT IS AN APPETITE STIMULANT
YOU WILL EAT MORE AND MORE AND...

Addictive Foods

Previous studies in animals conclude that highly processed foods, or foods with added fat or refined carbohydrates (like white flour and sugar) may be capable of triggering addictive-like eating behavior.[42] The brain reward centres light up with certain, especially sugary, foods. To some people this is simply an overwhelming desire – an addiction

Research suggests that we crave fatty and sugary foods when we are bored. This strengthens the theory that boredom is related to low levels of the stimulating brain chemical dopamine and that people try to boost this by eating fat and sugar if they cannot alleviate their boredom in some other way. Bored people do not eat nuts.

Overweight people make unhealthier food choices than lean people when presented with real food, even though both make similar selections when presented with hypothetical choices. The brain structure in obese people

---

[42] Erica M. Schulte, Nicole M. Avena, Ashley N. Gearhardt. Which Foods May Be Addictive? The Roles of Processing, Fat Content, and Glycemic Load. *PLOS ONE*, 2015; 10 (2): e0117959 DOI: 10.1371/journal.pone.0117959

Psst! Wanna Gain 269%

In the 1970s scientist Anthony Sclafani, in order to get otherwise normal rats to overeat, fed them an assortment of supermarket foods including Fruit Loops, chocolate-chip cookies, marshmallows and sweetened condensed milk in addition to their regular lab chow diet. The rats then virtually ignored the lab chow and overate the supermarket foods to extreme (morbid) obesity.[43] From memory they gained up to some 269% in weight.

Don't get jealous of the rats. You can do it too! Just buy all those center-aisle, packaged foods at the Supermarket and buy Heat and Eat meals.

Success Determined by Selecting "Likes"[44]

Dieters tend to adopt the wrong strategies, often planning to ditch their favorite foods and replace them with less-desirable options. Conversely, successful dieters focus on adding healthy foods - foods that they actually like. Opt for strategies that focus on including healthy foods in your diet and focus specifically on those healthy foods that you really enjoy eating.

Legumes and Pulses may help lose weight and keep it off

Eating one serving a day of beans, peas, chickpeas or lentils could contribute to modest weight loss.[45]

Nuts

A study of 273,000 participants who ate the most nuts not only had less weight gain than their nut-abstaining peers, but also enjoyed a 5 percent lower risk of becoming overweight or obese.[46]

But, avoid salted nuts. Salt is an appetite stimulant and it's very hard not to keep eating more and more.

ADDED SWEET
DON'T EAT

---

[43] Sclafani, A., & Springer, D. (1976). Dietary obesity in adult rats: Similarities to hypothalamic and human obesity syndromes. *Physiology & Behavior, 17*, 461-471.

[44] Saying "No" to Cake or "Yes" to Kale: Approach and Avoidance Strategies in Pursuit of Health Goals. *Psychology & Marketing*, 2016; 33 (8): 588 DOI: 10.1002/mar.20901

[45] Effects of dietary pulse consumption on body weight: a systematic review and meta-analysis of randomized controlled trials. *American Journal of Clinical Nutrition*, March 2016 DOI: 10.3945/ajcn.115.124677

[46] Loma Linda University Adventist Health Sciences Center

Sugar Beverages

- Soft drink, fruit punches contain large amounts of sugars and are associated with a greater magnitude of weight gain and an increased risk for development of type 2 diabetes[47]
- On any given day, half the people in the U.S. consume sugary drinks; 1 in 4 get at least 200 calories from such drinks; and 5% get at least 567 calories—equivalent to four cans of soda.[48]
- Sugary drinks (soda, energy, sports drinks) are the top calorie source in teens' diets (226 calories per day), beating out pizza (213 calories per day).[49]

The Obesity Surge: Excess sugar, carbs, not physical inactivity

Many people wrongly believe that obesity is entirely due to lack of exercise, a perception that is firmly rooted in junk food marketing.

Regular exercise is a key to staving off serious disease, such as diabetes, heart disease, and dementia but our calorie laden diets now generate more ill health than physical inactivity, alcohol, and smoking combined.

The prevalence of diabetes increases 11-fold for every 150 additional sugar calories consumed daily, compared with the equivalent amount of calories consumed as fat. And the evidence now suggests that carbs are no better.

Recent research indicates that cutting down on dietary carbohydrate, especially refined, is the single most effective approach for reducing all of the features of the metabolic syndrome and should be the primary strategy for treating diabetes, with benefits occurring even in the absence of weight loss.[50]

As noted, it is not just the one food type but *the overeating of all foods*. It is too simplistic to blame just one food. Overweight and obesity are multifactorial in this Obesogenic society.

---

[47] JAMA 2004;292

[48] Ogden CL, Kit BK, Carroll MD, Park S. Consumption of sugar drinks in the United States, 2005-2008<. *NCHS Data Brief*. 2011:1-8.

[49] National Cancer Institute. Mean Intake of Energy and Mean Contribution (kcal) of Various Foods Among US Population, by Age, NHANES 2005–06. Accessed June 21, 2012, http://riskfactor. cancer.gov/diet/foodsources/

[50] A. Malhotra, T. Noakes, S. Phinney. It is time to bust the myth of physical inactivity and obesity: you cannot outrun a bad diet. *British Journal of Sports Medicine*, 2015; DOI: 10.1136/ bjsports-2015-094911

CHAPTER 17

UNNATURAL

World War 2 (WW2) boosted the research into nutrition and the processing of foods. Since then over 85,000 chemicals have been invented, many of which have found their way into our foods and the food chain. Most are untested and only investigated when there is some catastrophe.

Obesity was only "noticed" in the 1980s which means people were certainly getting fatter for some time prior. The current vogue in some medical quarters is to blame our genes or our gut microbiome *but these have not altered.*

The only thing that has altered is the food we eat.

I contend that the graph of this current overweight-obesity epidemic would perfectly shadow the ingestion of processed foods - well close enough!

Processed, fast, pre-prepared, junk foods are full of these refined carbs and chemical additives and I think we simply cannot metabolize them.

Processed Cascade
The problem with foods that make people fat isn't all caused in that they have too many calories, but also, it's that they cause a cascade of reactions in the body that promote fat storage and make people overeat. Processed carbohydrates—foods like chips, sugar-soda/soft drinks, crackers/cakes/biscuits, and even white rice—digest quickly into sugar and increase levels of the hormone insulin.

It took humans millions of years to develop salivary amylase so as to digest grains (and get essential vitamins). In my book NEWTRITION I point out how an orange has some 70 micro-nutrients as well as its vitamin C. Humans can't make their own vitamin C, so we evolved to extract it from foods such as oranges (a deficiency resulted in scurvy). And I contend that the other 69 micro-nutrients in the orange help the vitamin C to be better metabolized or used by humans. Whereas we simply cannot "evolve" to metabolize these new chemicals invented in the last decades.

I also recounted the discovery of the first vitamin or 'vital amine', thiamine or vitamin B_1 which came from the husk of rice such that the Dutch Officers in Java in the nineteenth century developed Berri-berri (swollen hearts) and nerve conduction problems because, as officers, they were served the polished white rice – no husks. Whereas the other ranks, served the brown rice, remained healthy and well.

What Diet Foods to Eat

The alteration of natural food ratios, (high-fat, low-carbs, high-protein or whatever) should be regarded with utmost suspicion.

It is the ingestion of *unnatural foods i.e. processed,* which is the problem. Cutting out these refined carbs and processed foods is to be encouraged, but the replacing of complex carbs with fat, as in the Keto Diet, is no long-term lifestyle solution for you.

Eating an all-round balanced diet as per Newtrition Foods, eating less and intermittent fasting is the life-time answer.

Below is a list of processed foods some of which are so ubiquitous or advertised and marketed so cleverly that they appear healthy. It is not just the invention of these processed foods but their marketing, availability and affordability. They are three times cheaper than healthy food, taste delicious and are available 24 hours a day, seven days a week, home delivered or drive-thru.

The Fast Food Industry is not evil but neither does it have a conscience. They supply an insatiable demand. They have infiltrated august medical establishments, schools, sporting organizations and have nobbled the politicians such that medical reports are supressed, and threats made of with-drawl of political donations or mass unemployment in critical areas.

Governments will not legislate against bad food, it is up to you to eat healthy.

PROCESSED POISON: Ready to Eat: Heat and Eat[51]

By a gratifying coincidence, which confirms my observations and contentions, the first study as to the effects of ultra-processed foods on health was published online February 11 in *JAMA Internal Medicine*. The Findings from this prospective study of a large French cohort suggest for the first time, that an increased proportion of ultra-processed foods in the diet is associated with a higher risk of overall mortality. Ultra-processed foods were defined[52] as ready-to-eat or ready-to-heat formulations made mostly from ingredients usually combined with additives.

Study Summary

Ultra-processed foods usually contain "empty calories" and have a high caloric content with little nutritional value. They are low in fiber and high in carbohydrates, saturated fats, and salt. Usually, they contain food additives and contaminants that may be harmful to health, including some that may be carcinogenic, according to this study.

Consumption of ultra-processed foods -- such as mass-produced and packaged snacks, sugary drinks, breads, confectioneries, ready-made meals, and processed meats -- has increased during the past several decades and is associated with an overall unbalanced nutritional profile. Greater consumption of ultra-processed foods is linked to higher incidence of dyslipidaemia, obesity, hypertension, cancer, and other noncommunicable diseases, according to a growing body of evidence.

People often select ultra-processed foods because of their affordability, ease of preparation, and resistance to spoilage. Such foods are also highly marketed and are often prominently displayed in supermarkets.

Yet such convenience may come at a cost.

- Ultra-processed foods accounted for 29.1%±10.9% of total energy intake. (In other words some people diets eat >40% junk).
- Factors associated with intake of ultra-processed foods were younger age (45-64 years), mean proportion of food in weight, lower income, lower educational level, living alone, higher body mass index and lower physical activity level
- For every 10% increase in the proportion of ultra-processed foods consumed, there was a statistically significant, 14% greater risk for all-cause mortality.

---

[51] *JAMA Intern Med.* Published online February 11, 2019.[1]
[52] NOVA food classification system, u

- Investigators concluded that increased intake of ultra-processed foods was associated with an overall higher mortality risk, although overall nutritional quality of the diet may play a confounding role.
- Because ultra-processed foods are widely available, affordable, highly marketed, ready to eat, and have a long shelf life, consumers find them attractive.
- The increase in ultra-processed food consumption during the past several decades may result in a growing burden of mortality from noncommunicable diseases.
- Foods that have undergone high-temperature processing may contain carcinogenic neoformed contaminants such as acrylamide.
- Processed meat consumption may be carcinogenic for humans, with sufficient evidence for colorectal cancer and a positive association with stomach cancer.
- Ultra-processed foods often contain additives linked to health concerns, such as titanium dioxide associated with increased risk for chronic intestinal inflammation and carcinogenesis, and emulsifiers that change gut microbiota composition, promoting low-grade intestinal inflammation, enhancing cancer induction, and increasing risk for metabolic syndrome.
- Artificial sweeteners may affect microbiota and promote onset of type 2 diabetes and metabolic diseases.
- Packaging of ultra-processed foods may contain bisphenol and other chemicals with endocrine-disrupting properties.
- Epidemiologic studies suggest that endocrine disruptors are associated with increased risk for endocrine cancers, diabetes, obesity, and other metabolic diseases.

POISON: DO NOT EAT! – Well certainly minimize.
REFINED CARBS AND SIMPLE SUGARS (often called "added sugars")

Sugar: Table sugar/white sugar (aka sucrose; may be cane sugar or beet sugar)
Confectioner's sugar
Honey (Even though honey exists in nature and isn't refined, it is a pure sugar.)
Agave syrup
Corn syrup and high-fructose corn syrup
Brown sugar
Molasses
Maple syrup
Fructose
Brown rice syrup
Maltose
Glucose syrup
Tapioca syrup
Rice bran syrup
Malt syrup

Dextran
Sorghum
Treacle
Panela
Saccharose
Carob syrup
Dextrose, dextran, dextrin, maltodextrin
Fruit juice concentrates

Fruit Juices except for lemon/lime juice. Most fruit juices require special equipment to produce in significant quantities.

All Kinds of Flour including wheat, oat, legume (pea and bean), rice, and corn flours. 100% stone-ground, whole meal flours are less refined and not as unhealthy as other types of flours because they are not as finely ground and take longer to digest.

Instant/Refined Grains including instant hot cereals like instant oatmeal, white rice, polished rice, and instant rice

Refined Starches such as corn starch, potato starch, modified food starch–essentially any powdered ingredient with the word "starch" in it

Soft Drinks / Sodas

Foods High in Refined Carbs and Added Sugars

All desserts except whole fruit
Ice cream, sherbet, frozen yogurt,
Most breads
Many crackers (100% stone-ground whole grain crackers are less refined)
Cookies
Cakes
Muffins

Most pastas, noodles and couscous
Jelly (sugar-free varieties exist but it's much healthier to make your own with unsweetened gelatin and fresh fruit)
Jams and preserves

Pancakes
Waffles
Pies
Pastries
Candy
Chocolate (dark, milk and white). Baker's chocolate is unsweetened and is therefore an exception.
Breaded or battered foods
All doughs (phyllo, pie crust, etc)
Bagels
Pretzels
Pizza (flour in the dough)
Puddings and custards
Corn chips
Caramel corn and kettle corn
Most granola bars, power bars, energy bars (unless sugar-free).

Most cereals except for unsweetened, 100% whole grain cereals in which you can see the whole grains in their entirety with the naked eye (unsweetened muesli, rolled oats, or unsweetened puffed grain cereals are good examples)

Rice wrappers
Tortillas (unless 100% stone-ground whole grain)
Most rice cakes and corn cakes (unless 100% whole grain)

Panko crumbs
Croutons
Fried vegetable snacks like green beans and carrot chips (usually contain added dextrin)
Ketchup
Honey mustard
Most barbecue sauces
Check labels on salsa, tomato sauces, salad dressings and other jarred/canned sauces for sugar/sweeteners
Sweetened yogurts and other sweetened dairy products
Honey-roasted nuts
Sweetened sodas
Chocolate milk (and other sweetened milks)
Condensed milk
Hot cocoa
Most milk substitutes (almond milk, soy milk, oat milk, etc) because they usually have sugar added– read label first
Sweet wines and liquors

IF IT'S IN A CELLOPHANE WRAP

DON'T FALL FOR THE TRAP

IF IT COMES IN A PACKET

IT'S A COMMERCIAL RACKET

F.

EXERCISE
and
PHYSICAL
ACTIVITY

128 Dr Mileham Hayes

CHAPTER 18

PHYSICAL ACTIVITY: EXERCISE

Most guidelines for obesity management recommend high exercise volumes, at 150 to 250 minutes/week and up to 60 minutes/day of moderate-intensity aerobic exercise. However, few people meet these guidelines.

The Good News
The good news is you can do this 30 minutes a day in six 5minute bursts.

The Even Better News
Modern research has found just 40 seconds three times a week is enough and that 40 seconds of SIT (see below) is the equivalent of running for 45 minutes.

Definitions
The exercise 'Industry' has now come up with numerous confusing permutations and combinations often referred to by their abbreviations but without the following explanations:
HIIT: High Intensity Interval Training - short bursts of demanding exercise interspersed with short rests
HIRT: the same, but with resistance training
HIFT: the functional version, designed to prepare you for any movement
MCIT or **MOD**: Moderate-Intensity Continuous Training
LISS: Low-Intensity Steady-State exercise, even a gentle stroll can now, technically, count and be considered a productive fat-loss session
HIIPA: High Intensity Incidental Physical Activity. Now touted as a simple way to push your body into healthy adaptation without disrupting your daily schedule. Changes recommended include using the stairs, carrying the shopping for 100 to 200 meters – or, if you walk at a low pace, accelerating to the point that you find it hard to speak.
SIT: Sprint Interval Training

Exercise is not very efficient for losing weight but is essential: Five times more energy is needed to get rid of fat than to get rid of muscle and so the body resists fat loss. 30 minutes of jogging or swimming may burn off 350 cals but it is much easier to consume 350 less calories by not drinking soda / soft drinks or non-hungry junk food eating.

From 2001 to 2009 Americans increased their exercise but obesity increased. You have to also reduce your calories!

Exercise, however, does help weight loss and its profound other benefits and should be part of any weight loss program. In a study published in *JAMA Network Open*, they asked more than 315,000 U.S. adults — between ages 50 and 71 — and their activity at four different points in their lives: when they were 15-18 years, 19-29 years, 35-39 years and 40-61 years.

People who said they exercised anywhere from two to eight hours a week at each time period had a 29% to 36% lower risk of dying from any cause during the study's 20-year period, compared to people who rarely or never exercised. They also lowered their risk of dying from heart disease by up to 42% and cancer by up to 14% compared to inactive people. The more people exercised, the greater their risk reductions.

SIT Best: Interval Training May Be Best for Weight Loss[53]

The latest research suggests Interval training may result in greater weight loss than continuous exercise, with sprint interval training (SIT) the most effective, say researchers, who say interval training also may be easier for obese and older individuals to perform. Interval training "seems to promote many physiological changes that might favor long-term weight loss.

Previous studies have shown that interval training is able to promote upregulation of important enzymes associated with fat degradation, which occurs to a greater extent than with moderate-intensity continuous exercise.

Interval training was associated with a reduction in total absolute fat mass that was more than 28% greater than that seen with MOD, with the greatest reductions seen with SIT.

The advantage of interval training is that it can be performed by almost everyone, but participants have to know how to adapt it and have in mind that 'intensity' is calculated individually

Research found that both interval training and MOD were associated with significant reductions in total body fat percentage, at –1.50% and –1.44%,

---

[53] *Br J Sports Med.* Published online February 14, 2019

respectively. Both forms of training were also linked to significant reductions in total absolute fat mass, at –1.58 kg for interval training. However, interval training was associated with a significantly greater reduction in total absolute fat mass versus MOD, at a relative reduction of –2.28 kg, or 28.5%.

In subgroup analyses, SIT was associated with even greater reductions in total absolute fat mass versus MOD, at –3.22 kg.

MOD, HITT or SIT[54]

Interval training may have the potential to promote weight loss as it has some benefits similar to moderate-intensity continuous training (MOD) while requiring less time. MOD is typically defined as continuous effort that elicits 55%–70% of the maximal heart rate (HRmax) or promotes oxygen consumption equivalent to 40%–60% of the maximum O_2 consumption. Interval training is an intermittent period of effort interspersed by recovery period; the two most common types of interval training are high-intensity interval training (HIIT) and sprint interval training (SIT). HIIT requires 'near maximal' efforts performed at a heart rate (HR) ≥80% of the HRmax. Even more intense exercise, SITs are efforts performed at intensities equal or superior to the one that elicited a peak O_2 consumption which included 'all-out' efforts.

Interval training was associated with a reduction in total absolute fat mass that was more than 28% greater than that seen with MOD, with the greatest reductions seen with SIT.

Interval training can be performed by almost everyone, but it has to be adapted by the individual and 'intensity' is calculated individually. Whereas most guidelines for obesity management recommend high exercise volumes, at 150 to 250 minutes/week and up to 60 minutes/day of moderate-intensity aerobic exercise but most people cannot achieve this.

---

[54] Is interval training the magic bullet for fat loss? A systematic review and meta-analysis comparing moderate-intensity continuous training with high-intensity interval training (HIIT). February 14, 2019, British Journal of Sports Medicine http://dx.doi.org/10.1136/bjsports-2018-099928

Fastest and Most Efficient: 20secs x2, x3times a week) - Recommended
Perhaps the most efficient regime, if you are healthy, is two sessions of 20 seconds of stationary cycling as fast as possible (40 seconds in toto) three times a week reduced muscle glycogen by 24% and stimulated the genes which improved overall CVS health. Interval training is able to promote upregulation of important enzymes associated with fat degradation, which occurs to a greater extent than with moderate-intensity continuous exercise.

Five weeks later aerobic fitness had improved by an average of 11% which reduces heart disease by 20%.

To achieve the same result (of glycogen depletion) it would be necessary to run for 45 minutes.

Slim 4 Life recommends SIT and HIIPA
i.e. A combination of 40 seconds exercise bike three times a week
and
Incidental Physical Activity – walking fast, taking the stairs until you puff.
Using the shopping for resistance weight training.

Psychological and behavioral responses to interval and continuous exercise[55]
Psychological responses to, and preferences for, moderate-intensity continuous training (MICT), high-intensity interval training (HIIT), and sprint interval training (SIT) among inactive adults were studied as well as the relationships between affect, enjoyment, exercise preferences, and subsequent exercise behavior over a 4-wk follow-up period.

This study provides new evidence that a single session of HIIT and SIT can be as enjoyable and preferable as MICT among inactive individuals and that there may be differences in the exercise affect-behavior relationship between interval and continuous exercise.

Strenuous and prolonged animal running experiment[56] suggests that intense exercise might change the workings of certain neurons in ways that could have

---

[55] Med Sci Sports Exerc. 2018 Oct;50(10):2110-2121. doi: 10.1249/MSS.0000000000001671.
Psychological and Behavioral Responses to Interval and Continuous Exercise.
[56] Cellular and synaptic reorganization of arcuate NPY/AgRP and POMC neurons after exercise. Molecular Metabolism, Volume 18, December 2018, Pages 107-119 https://doi.org/10.1016/j.molmet.2018.08.011

beneficial effects on appetite and metabolism.

The closest human equivalent I know that mimics this regime is marathon running – and I don't think any marathon runner would be reading this book.

Obviously, you should get medical clearance before proceeding. For a healthy young man, a sprint probably involves running at high velocities, but for a frail elder, slow walking might be enough. For individuals who have knee problems and are not able to run, you can cycle or even swim. If you have heart disease, you can walk at a controlled intensity. But, as above, a stationary bike would seem the overall best choice.

Exercise is important especially for maintaining weight loss long-term.

One of its most useful contributions is that it minimizes the increases in hunger experienced from dieting. It does not cause an increase in hunger to the same extent as dieting, despite, if and when, it burns off the same reduction in calories. In fact, hunger is reduced when exercising intensely[57], which may help to stave off hunger pangs while increasing the energy deficit.

The effect of exercise for maintaining weight loss was also recently highlighted with participants from the US televised weight loss competition, *The Biggest Loser*. The tracking of participants for six years after the show revealed that the people who maintained their weight loss had increased their physical activity by 160 percent. Whereas those who regained their lost weight had only increased physical activity by 34 percent[58].

As pointed out in the last chapter, exercise has been touted by the soda-soft drink and fast-food industries as the healthy way to lose weight. They infiltrate and donate to sports clubs and such to get their brand names up and their products installed. They promote the false images with some paid athlete or model drinking a cola, eating a health bar, jogging or in a gym that if you exercise you to will be slim like their product consuming models.

This is just a cynical exploitation. The truth is the direct opposite.

---

[57] Proceedings of the Nutrition Society Volume 73, Issue 2 May 2014 , pp. 352-358 Creating an acute energy deficit without stimulating compensatory increases in appetite: is there an optimal exercise protocol? Kevin Deighton and David J Stensel
https://doi.org/10.1017/S002966511400007XPublished online: 09 April 201
[58] Obesity volume25, Issue11 November 2017 Pages 1838-1843

The people who drink sugary drinks and eat fast foods are invariably overweight. The athlete or model being paid $millions to endorse their product would have a very healthy diet to remain slim and to keep people eating their Fast Food they claim exercise will do it and that their high-calorie junk is not the cause.

The Gym Junkie Mistake
While exercise is important it far less efficient than reducing calories for losing weight. Both low and high intensity exercise regimes led to the same weight and waist reduction. Losing weight is a strict fitness regime wherein, to be successful, like any achievement, you have to record your performance every day and keep improving. Regular monitoring is also the key to how Weight Watchers achieves success.

It is a curious contradiction when Gym Junkies can find an hour or more, not forgetting the drive, parking, showers, but then complain there is not enough time to cook – where they can actually control their calories. And where they become obsessed with gym workout routines but are in denial as to the calories they ingest and often their nutrition includes dubious gym supplements.

That said in Cuba in the 1990s there was no real motorized transport so free bicycles were provided. Food was also scarce and rationed. So, the population exercised more, ate less, lost 5.5 kg on average while diabetes dropped and heart disease by 53% only to relapse to the previous health problems when the crisis was over Similarly, elsewhere it is pointed out how the UK was never healthier when a similar crisis was imposed by WW2.

In 2013, the *International Journal of Epidemiology* detailed the evidence that physical activity is not key to losing weight. Since then multiple lines of evidence lead to the conclusion that an increase in physical activity is offset by an increase in calorie intake, unless conscious effort is made to limit that compensatory response. In addition, it has been found that the body adapts to higher activity levels changing the metabolism and fewer calories are burned.
Physical activity generally decreases along with age. Participants whose total step count grew by more than 2,000 steps during the follow-up period, maintained their BMI at the same level throughout the years. In contrast, BMI increased for those whose step count stayed at the same level or decreased[59].

---

[59] University of Jyväskylä Sep 2017

Weight training appears key to controlling belly fat as we age
Healthy men who did 20 minutes of daily weight training had less increase in age-related abdominal fat compared with men who spent the same time doing aerobic activities. This is due to sarcopaenia, loss of muscle mass, as we age.

10,000 Steps (Try 12,000)
There is no evidence to support this popular recommendation. It was a marketing strategy to sell step counters. It began with Japanese walking clubs and a business slogan 30+ years ago. And promoted in the lead-up to the 1964 Tokyo Olympics and to sell pedometers. Then the concept was revisited by Australian researchers in 2001 to encourage people to be more active.

While 10,000 steps/day appears to be a reasonable goal for daily activity for apparently healthy adults and studies are emerging documenting the health benefits of attaining similar levels, preliminary evidence suggests that it may not be sustainable for some groups, including older adults and those living with chronic diseases. Another concern about using 10 000 steps/day as a universal step goal is that it is probably too low for children, an important target population in the war against obesity. Based on currently available evidence, it has been proposed the following preliminary indices be used to classify pedometer-determined physical activity in healthy adults[60]:

(i)   <5000 steps/day may be used as a 'sedentary lifestyle index';

(ii)   5000–7499 steps/day is typical of daily activity excluding sports/exercise and might be considered 'low active';

(iii)   7500–9999 likely includes some volitional activities (and/or elevated occupational activity demands) and might be considered 'somewhat active'; and

(iv)   ≥10 000 steps/day indicates the point that should be used to classify individuals as 'active'. Individuals who take >12 500 steps/day are likely to be classified as 'highly active' and maintain weight loss.

Slim 4 Life recommends SIT but if you want to walk short bursts of 5 minutes. 6x5 = 30 minutes a day = 150 minutes a week are as good as continuous.

---

[60] Sports Medicine January 2004, Volume 34, Issue 1, pp 1–8| Cite as
How Many Steps/Day Are Enough? Preliminary Pedometer Indices for Public Health

The latest research recommends 12,000 steps a day to maintain weight loss. Viz:

- The weight-loss maintainer group demonstrated significantly higher levels of steps per day (12,000 steps per day) compared to participants at a normal body weight (9,000 steps per day) and participants with overweight/obesity (6,500 steps per day).[61]

Tips

1. Make exercise an important priority
2. Select best time: Early morning, after work, evening. No commitment that can make you miss or cancel
3. Ensure adequate sleep and contented mood
4. Shorten workouts – SIT or 6x5 x 30 min brisk walking or 12,000 steps
5. Use distractions: Music, exercise apps, videos, podcasts, radio
6. Set precise 4 week goals e.g. Lengthen distance decrease time
7. Plan ahead and stick to it
8. Exercise with a companion
9. Pay yourself

Most Importantly

As you lose weight your Metabolic Rate falls and you then have to do more exercise.

IF YOU ARE BREATHING HARD

YOU HAVE BEEN EXERCISING EFFICIENTLY –

MUSCLES ARE BEING TONED

Self-Deception and Accelerometers[62]

Analysis has found that higher levels of physical activity are associated with lower adiposity whether measured by BMI, % body fat, or waist circumference but were twice as strong when measured by accelerometers instead of estimated from self-report which suggests that people with higher adiposity are less accurate in assessing how much activity they take.

---

[61] Obesity March 2019

[62] *BMJ Open* doi:10.1136/bmjopen-2018-024206.

Move more and sit less

The new USA physical-activity guidelines were updated in 2018 for the first time since 2008, and they still urge adults to do 75 minutes of vigorous (or 150 minutes of moderate) aerobic activity each week, plus muscle-strengthening sessions like weight-lifting or yoga twice a week. But only 23% of Americans do so, and a recent study found that a quarter of American adults sit for more than eight hours per day. But recent research suggests that any daily activity rather than formal exercises provide longevity benefits.

In a study of older women published last year in the *Journal of the American Geriatrics Society*, with each 30-minute chunk of light activities like these, people lowered their risk of dying early by 12% compared to their more sedentary peers. And a 2018 study found that among older men, each additional half hour of light physical activity, such as walking or gardening, slashed their risk of early death by 17%. The addition of a simpler imperative to the guidelines

The Gym Scam:

When the Fast Food Industry blamed lack of exercise for obesity and that exercise would fix it, gyms erupted throughout the Western world promising the defined body…at 5 hours intensive exercise a week plus a strict diet and worth & $billion a year. People joined gyms to lose weight but they quit because they didn't – often leaving their paid up subscriptions for the gym owners to collect for doing nothing.

It has been found (Prof Wilkins) that people who exercise intensively then just sit around for the rest of the day. He feels this is an evolutionary compensation wherein animals would never expend unnecessary energy.

The exercise phenomenon that morphed into the gym cult began in Muscle Beach Los Angeles in the 1970s especially with Richard Simmons who lost 100lb. Having been obese himself he understood the obese and offered more than a simple workout. He offered them self-respect and self-worth.

Lycra, gym gear, supplements boomed.

Jane Fonda revolutionized it for women and transformed the gym culture

Gyms became losing weight centres.

Losing weight became the business model for the gym industry. Ingenuous.

The food industry reinforced it that 'moving more is the way to get thin' i.e. you can still eat fast food. They, Coke, McDonald's and Cadburys, were amongst the biggest sponsors of the 2012 Olympic Games with the biggest McDonald's in the World. Fast Food Companies sponsor and associate themselves with sport. Their message is that their food or drink is fine as long as you exercise. They corrupt the "Calories In = Calories out equations" claiming they contribute little to the input whilst exercise burns off the calories out: If you do enough exercise you can do what you like.

Their sponsorship of sport and advocation of exercise, allows them to claim they are 'part of the solution'. This nobbles legislation against their advertising and sponsorship.

G.

HINTS, TRICKS and GOOD ADVICE

CHAPTER 19

HINTS, TRICKS and GOOD ADVICE

Habits of The Most Successful Slimmers
These habits may not be obvious as their practitioners seldom make a big issue as to their behavior(s), or it has been so entrenched that it is familiar second nature and people accept this as their normal manner of conduct e.g. "(S)he eats like a bird" of persons we all know as not eating much and we accept their actions as 'just being them'. These twelve daily habits define some of the best-looking people:

1. Total ruthless dedication to their plan
2. Daily control and continuance. Never give up
3. Emancipation not deprivation
4. The best foods (Newtrition Super-Mediterranean)
5. Never feeling full. Always leaving something on the plate
6. Interest in health. Pride in appearance
7. Aerobic and Resistance exercise
8. Always alternatives to eating (exercise or occupation)
9. Portion control
10. No processed foods. No sugar or refined carbs
11. Dedication, Determination, Discipline, Resolve and Restraint
12. Anti-Disillusionment strategies

HINTS
- Re-set your volume control. Eat smaller portions. Think thin: Think small volumes of the food you eat
- While calories and volume are not the same, they are if you eat high-nutrition foods. If we eat greater volumes they fill us more
- Eat less, just two days a week
- Portion Distortion: From 1960 - 2012 portion sizes increased > x 10 times for coke and 100 cals for fries, hamburgers
- You only need 20 more cals a day to gain weight and 100cals extra a day to become obese
- People do not notice an extra 1000cals a day. "Insensible eating" Monitor!
- Eat with someone who eats small amounts – social modeling

- Never eat everything on your plate. Leave a third. Never eat until you feel 'full'
- Intermittent fasts – 600cal days x twice a week. Otherwise, rest of week, eat as before
- Eating 600 calories a day less for men from 2,400 to 1,800 calories gave better results (fat 2.3 vs 1.3% in six months)
- Think more vegetarian who are the slimmest people but not in twin studies (one eats meat). So, Lifestyle also helps.
- Stick to the Newtrition Foods (emphasizing vegetarian). Don't worry about % of protein, carbohydrate or fats
- Otherwise measure Calories av = < 1800 Cals / day for men, <1,500 Cals /day for women
- This, along with a near fresh vegetarian / fish diet, is the secret of most of the world's longest living people
- Get your mind made up, determined and set to go. No excuses, no stress, no competing interests
- Ensure some 'my time' to get away, review and plan each week
- Get help. Enlist a partner to monitor and support
- Avoid the 'Supermarket' and processed foods especially sugar, fats and unrefined carbohydrates
- Compensate for junk by buying the best as a substitution reward
- Identify hi-Cal junk foods and avoid
- Whole fruit and small half-hand-full nuts for snacks
- Exercise - the type doesn't matter (SIT best) but you must also eat less. Eating less is far more efficient than exercise
- Beware the exercise 'Entitlement Trap' that exercise 'justifies' more food. Exercise can weaken self-control
- No unearned 'rewards'. Treats must be earned e.g. after a sustained minimum 3 kg loss. But then resume eating less
- To lose - No booze
- Measure waist circumference
- Weigh daily
- Diet diary-Phone App excellent help – but record *everything*
- Everyone falls off the wagon, gets disillusioned, but this should be a key to get going again
- You will hit the wall and feel lousy at six weeks or 10% weight loss. Be warned! Continue! Increase exercise.

- Your body will hit its default values - the weights you were stuck on as you gained and will resist change. Continue
- Do not have unreal expectations. Don't feel sorry for yourself – the lean also have to work at it too
- Think long term: 250 g loss a week = 13 kg a year = 28.6lb or 2 stone a year. (Would you like to gain that?)
- Put up a photo of someone you want to look like
- Don't shop when hungry – if you don't buy it you can't eat it. Remember Mother Hubbard – she was lean
- Identify triggers or cravings – make plans to avoid. Identify non-hungry eating
- People who don't lose underestimate the food they eat by 47% to 67% and overestimate activity by 40% to 51%
- Fat people unconsciously snack.
- Don't open the fridge and graze. Hide snacks lower shelf at back
- Make eating formal, pleasant and slow. No mindless snacking in front of TV. Minimize restaurants and Takeaways.
- People ate twice the amount of M&Ms if they were labeled 'lite'. Don't believe "Lite, No sugar, Sugar reduced, Low Fat"
- Don't start unless and until you are absolutely resolved and committed with no excuses
- Restricting dietary fat can lead to greater body fat loss than carb restriction
- Clear the kitchen bench of everything but the fruit bowl
- Catch the bus or train. Use the stairs.
- Vegans have the lowest BMI, then vegetarians but not by all that much in identical twin studies there was only a 1.5kg difference. Vegans usually have a stricter Lifestyle.
- People keenly interested in their food are usually interested in their health and therefore their weight too
- When selecting foods in a sequence (e.g., at a buffet or on a food ordering website), individuals are influenced by the first item they see and tend to make their subsequent food choices on the basis of this first item. This notion can be utilized to nudge individuals into consuming less food overall. In contrast to what one might intuitively assume, when an indulgent dish is the first item, lower-calorie dishes are subsequently chosen, and overall caloric consumption is lower and vice versa. They

didn't even have to eat the treat first; just knowing they had selected it was enough to trigger a change.[63]

- Medicine has vogues, if not fads, and the latest vogue is the Gut microbiome or microbes. While this plays as yet an unknown but important place, it is not the complete multifactorial answer
- Scientists from several different laboratories found that sweet, bitter, and other taste receptors found in the mouth also exist in the gut — so the gut literally does taste food after it is consumed. Carbohydrates can thus be preferred and while the palatability of fat has taste and post-ingestion components as well, it also includes mouth feel sensations such as creamy texture
- We can blame our genes, we can blame our gut but, if we are to lose weight, we have to eat smaller amounts (less calories) and avoid processed foods

Information is Power

No one else can provide you with the willpower. However, 'Information is power' which may give you an understanding of the problem and this recent overweight-obesity phenomenon and provide you with the facts to reinforce your resolve and not the dreams and scams of the fad diets that will lead you up the garden path… to the fat farm.

Clear the kitchen bench of everything but the fruit bowl

Women who had breakfast cereal sitting on their counters weighed 20lbs (9kg) more than their neighbors who didn't, and those with soft drinks sitting out weighed 24 to 26lbs (11–12kg) more. Those who had a fruit bowl weighed about 13lbs (6kg) less.

Eat Small and Wait

It takes some 20 minutes for the food to descend to that part of our intestines to register feeling full / satisfied.

Overeating Healthy Food

When people eat what they consider healthy food, they eat more than the recommended serving size as they associate "healthy" with less filling.

---

[63] *Journal of Experimental Psychology: Applied.* Advance online publication. http://dx.doi. org/10.1037/xap0000210

Large Tables - Smaller Portions
To eat less serve food in small portions and on large tables.

Eating vs. Exercise
It takes 90 minutes to exercise off 2 minutes of eating

Bus and tram users are slimmer than car drivers
A study of more than 150,000 commuters, aged 49 to 69 from the U.K., who used public transportation, tended to have a lower body mass and a reduced percentage of body fat compared with those who drove to work.
It is reasoned that physical activity during commuting has health benefits even if its intensity is moderate and the commuting does not cause high heart rate and sweating.

Water Boarding
Drinking 500 ml of water at half an hour before eating main meals may help obese adults to lose weight. Those who reported preloading before all three main meals in the day reported a loss of 4.3kg (9.48lbs) over the 12 weeks, whereas those who only preloaded once, or not at all, only lost an average of 0.8kg (1.76lbs).

To keep it off, do not eat processed foods
This simplistic equation has been criticized by the gut microbiome (bacteria) enthusiasts, but I have been struck by documentaries of a white boy and his Bushman (of the Kalahari Desert) friend who met again after a 40year gap. The Bushman, now in his 60s had exactly the same lean figure and physique. He still ran and hunted and ate non-processed food. While gut bacteria obviously play a part, the type and amount of food and the amount of exercise still make this advice (eat natural foods, not processed) basically sensible. Intermittent fasting also seems to help.

All Pigs are equal, but some pigs are more equal than others.
George Orwell, Animal Farm

We are not all created equal and one person can eat a kilogram of food and will put on a kilogram while another will hardly gain any weight. This is due both to genetics and our gut flora (microbes) but while we can blame our genes and microbes, if you overeat and eat junk you will gain weight. Genetics and gut bugs do not completely explain the modern epidemic of obesity: Processed - junk food, increased intake and sedentary lifestyles also contribute. The Fast Food Industry spends $Trillions lobbying Governments such that medical evidence is ignored or buried, and junk food is either labeled 'healthy' or packaged to seduce you into thinking it is.

You Are What You Think You Eat[64]

Despite eating the same breakfast, made from the same ingredients, people consumed more calories throughout the day when they believed that one of the breakfasts was less than the other. When the participants believed that their omelette was smaller, they reported themselves to be significantly hungrier after two hours, they consumed significantly more of a pasta lunch and, in total, consumed significantly more calories throughout the day than when the same participants believed that they were eating a larger omelette.

Underweight people pay greater attention to natural foods and overweight people to processed foods[65].

The Thrifty 'Fat' Gene[66]

The Thrifty Fat gene Hypothesis proposes that the ability to store fat provided an evolutionary advantage when food could be scarce. The corollary is that the body perceives weight loss as dysfunctional and strives to correct it by promoting hunger and weight regain. But what was an advantage is now a disadvantage.

There is no doubt that there are some people who are genetically programmed to put on weight or lay down fat more "efficiently" than others. This has been referred to, in broad, as the Thrifty Gene when it is probably a number of genes. Various claims are made from some 127 to 6,000 genes which are claimed can account for some 40% difference in weight. These people were arguably genetically superior in the early days of human existence when famines, droughts, floods, ice-ages, locust plagues and what-have-you, caused forced, long migrations. These were survival genes against famine. Fat was rare and essential; the fat part of any animal e.g. the Pope's Nose was thus always reserved for the best hunter to provide him with fat (energy) reserves, so he could continue hunting. Wild animals always eat the liver first as it is protein dense. However, it was the

[64] British Psychological Society (BPS). "You are what you think you eat." ScienceDaily September 2017. <www.sciencedaily.com/releases/2017/09/170907104304.htm>.
[65] A neural signature of food semantics is associated with body-mass index. *Biological Psychology*, 2017; DOI: 10.1016/j.biopsycho.2017.09.001
[66] Yale J Biol Med, 2014;87:99-112

people with this Thrifty Gene who laid down fat more easily or efficiently, that most survived these enforced migrations. They didn't need 'fattening-up'. When they ate, they put on more fat than most and they survived the bad times. This 'fat gene' predisposes perhaps 20% of people to be overweight / obese. This is a profound medical problem making losing weight much harder; some experts feel, impossible.

In the early 70s I was attached to what was arguably one of the first obesity clinics in the world at an Edinburgh Hospital and we were very surprised when one of our very low-calorie patient's graph, which had been plummeting, suddenly spiked significantly. She was meticulously supervised and observed 24 hours a day to make sure she did not access any food. Her sudden significant weight gain was all due to having milk in her tea! While there may be other metabolic pathways yet to be discovered, I have always thought these people are 'super-absorbers'. They put on 90% (+) of what they eat whereas a skinny person may not put on much or any fat at all. However, the more one eats the more efficient absorption becomes. Recent research implicates our gut flora, our gut microbiome of our own bacteria as contributing but there would seem a lot of research yet to be done.

Fattening up for migration is not unique to humans. Birds who still do annual incredibly long migrations of thousands and thousands of miles, feed up until they are super-fat. However, if and when they arrive without being able to eat (flying over oceans) they are skinny without any body fat left. Today, however, these erstwhile efficient human 'fat absorbers' are at a much greater risk as there are no famines and no long migrations, and fat making processed-food is available 24 hours a day, seven days a week, 365 days a year and we will deliver it plus a giant fructose sweetened cola to your TV chair. Now our only 'migration' is to a Drive-Thru Hamburger stand (with large fries and cola). In this food toxic environment, we are all at risk: We all run the risk of accepting larger portions and servings as 'good value', eating everything we have paid for, even if we are not hungry, and eating processed food because it is cheap, easy and delicious. And so, unlike the Bushmen of the Kahalari who remain slim, we think it is 'normal' to gain weight as we age.

H

OMG

150 Dr Mileham Hayes

CHAPTER 20

OMG: THE WRONG FOOD

WE ARE GETTING FATTER AND FATTER

There is no greater daily available pleasure reward than food, especially food manipulated to hit the bliss point. The brain reward-centers light up with certain, especially sugary / sweet foods. To some people this is simply an overwhelming desire – an addiction.

Studies in animals conclude that highly processed foods, or foods with added fat or refined carbohydrates (like white flour and sugar) and highly processed foods like chocolate, pizza and French fries are among the most addictive. Unprocessed foods, with no added fat or refined carbohydrates like brown rice and salmon, were not associated with addictive-like eating behavior.

Research suggests that we crave fatty and sugary foods when we are bored. This strengthens the theory that boredom is related to low levels of the stimulating brain chemical dopamine and that people try to boost this by eating fat and sugar if they cannot alleviate their boredom in some other way.

Looks Good to Me
Overweight people make unhealthier food choices than lean people when presented with real food, even though both make similar selections when presented with hypothetical choices.

Fastest Fat Gains
There is a tribe in Africa where the unmarried young men try to gain weight as the one who gains the most weight in the allocated time gets the pick of a marriage mate. The men achieve this by lying down, doing no exercise and drinking as much full cream milk as possible.

The woman who held most distance world swimming records ate cheese-cake to put on fat most quickly to insulate her against the cold of the English Channel.

Russian Circus Lions and Processed Food

Not Just Us: In 2017 in Russia it was found performing circus lions were now obese because they were being fed a junk food diet to save money.

The Wrong Food

Since World War 2 over 85,000 synthetic chemicals have been introduced many of which find their way into the associated phenomenon of processed, ultra-processed and additive foods.

We are not only eating too much but too much of this new junk, processed food. Many of these additives are untested and, in any event, we simply have not had time to evolve to metabolize them: We can't process the processed foods.

Healthiest

The British and the Cubans have never been healthier as when food rationing was enforced (WW2 and the USA Embargo).

Who's Dieting?

On any given day 70% of women will be dieting and 80% will try to lose weight at least once this year while 60% feel they have difficulty controlling their weight. 60% of overweight women are trying to lose weight but so are 35% of those who are not overweight. Women are secretive about weight worry and control methods.

As to men, 25% are trying to lose weight, 40% will try to lose weight at least once this year, 33% of overweight men do not want to lose weight.

Wider Seats, Reinforced Operating Tables

The number of Americans who are too grossly overweight to fit into an airline seats has increased by 350% in 30 years. Operating tables now have to be made stronger to take the weight of the fatter population.

Nutrition

Eat only the **Newtrtion Super-Mediterranean foods.** These foods are evidenced to confer best health benefits and optimize longevity

Human nutrition science has historically either focused on a single-nutrient approach such as the absence of vitamin C causing scurvy or to blame fat, carbohydrates or sugar, in isolation, as causes of the obesity crisis. But, in reality, todays modern nutrition-related diseases are driven by an overabundance of food, an evolved fondness for foods containing particular blends of nutrients (e,g, chocolate) and clever marketing by the packaged food industry exploiting these preferences.

Health Foods
If it's labeled 'healthy' then what are fresh fruit and vegetables?
Be wary of other 'health' foods: Some 'health' smoothies contain over 500 calories!

There also now seems that there is no sensible, middle road. The health-exercisers and the Diet Zealots zeal is frankly cult-like and off-putting. Their regimes are incredible self-obsessed, anti-social rituals which are not "normal" or necessary. If that's what it takes to lose weight and get fit, no wonder many of us give up.

Fresh vs Processed
The people who live longest are peasant societies where there is no processed foods but fresh every-day home grown vegetables, herbs and fruit, little meat, olive oil and not much transport - they walk.

And they are not obese.

I looked at the breakfast cereal of some friends who are dedicated Walkers: "Wholegrain muesli with burnt fig, with almonds dipped in honey and rolled in cinnamon" and from "Farmer Jack" or some similar reassuring-sounding primary producer. It was in a superb attractive 'organic' presentation urging us to "want me, eat me, love me" and it *was* delicious!

But it was in a package and when I looked at the ingredients per 100grams (the best measure) and the sugar content (yes honey is sugar) it was 17.3g. No wonder it tasted delicious - the recommended g/100g for sugar is <4g. This "healthy" breakfast muesli was four times more than medically recommended) and it was 1880kj per 100grams or 450calories per 3.5 ounces.

I think it was a genuine attempt to make a healthier muesli and that most are a lot, lot worse but...it still comes in a package and it's processed and while we try

to do the right healthy thing and buy these beautifully attractive breakfast cereals proclaiming or insinuating how healthy they are, they are still processed foods.
The breakfast cereal racket began with Dr Kellog and the Seventh Day Adventist Church. Kellog obviously thought his corn flakes were healthy - so healthy in fact that he claimed they would "cure masturbation". But at least he was a qualified medical practitioner and there was some basis for his (incorrect) beliefs. However, the unqualified founder of the Seventh Day Adventists had a "vision", presumably of the Lord, who told her she should not smoke (good!), drink alcohol (a little wine actually may be beneficial) and not eat meat (stupid and wrong). He also told her to go to Australia and so the vegetarian breakfast cereal industry was born.

She is credited with claiming "Breakfast is the most important meal of the day" also incredibly wrong but hey! Sales of Corn Flakes and Weet Bix boomed! Just add processed refined sugar in excess to these processes and refined factory wheat flakes and they are almost palatable - unless you are gluten-sensitive.

Maybe, if you think about it, breakfast cereals may be the original cause of this obesity epidemic - I mean overdosing on sugar in the morning?

In 2019, in fact, research found that breakfast was not necessary and people who ate breakfast weighed more.

But, in addition, the bacon sales were dropping, so Sigmund Freud's nephew was hired by the USA bacon producers to reinforce the (false) message that breakfast was indeed the most important meal of the day by conning 5,000 doctors to agree and bacon sales boomed.

But hey! Bacon with nitrites and all processed meats are implicated in causing cancer of the colon but sales of it and sugar breakfast cereals are booming!

Nutritionists and dietitians, funded by the Seventh Day Adventist church, still endorse this scientifically, medical falsehood.

And we are getting fatter and fatter and fatter.

Now if you feel like breakfast, and the manual or farm workers of old certainly did and needed it, then eat it! But fresh fruit, berries, nuts and plain, unsweetened yogurt (I give the recipe for "the World's Best Breakfast" in NEWTRITION) are incredibly better for you or, at least, not as injurious as processed foods with sugar, no matter how much they are promoted as healthy by the factory.

Breakfast cereals, ham, bacon and sausages with preservatives, are processed foods.

All this rant is but to get across to you how insidious and all pervasive the Fast Food Industry is. How it often basks behind a false halo of being health food, spends $billions on advertising and nobbling politicians to invade every aspect and corner of our lives unless, it would seem, we become health-nut zealots.

Surely there is a sensible middle road?

Yes, there is, but we also have to be informed, on guard, disciplined and resolved.

BAD FOODS
Sugar Beverages
* * Soft drink, fruit punches contain large amounts of readily absorbable sugars and are associated with a greater magnitude of weight gain and an increased risk for development of type 2 diabetes
    * On any given day, half the people in the U.S. consume sugary drinks; 1 in 4 get at least 200 calories from such drinks; and 5% get at least 567 calories—equivalent to four cans.
    * Sugary drinks (soda, energy, sports drinks) are the top calorie source in teens' diets (226 calories per day), beating out pizza (213 calories per day).

Excess sugar and refined carbs, not physical inactivity, are behind the surge in obesity

Many people wrongly believe that obesity is entirely due to lack of exercise, a perception that is firmly rooted in corporate marketing. Regular exercise is a help to staving off serious disease, such as diabetes, heart disease, and dementia but our calorie laden diets now generate more ill health than physical inactivity, alcohol, and smoking combined.

As already pointed out the public relations tactics of the food industry are "chillingly similar to those of Big Tobacco," used to convince the public that smoking was not linked to lung cancer.

Sugar calories promote fat storage and hunger. Fat calories induce fullness or satiation. The prevalence of diabetes increases 11-fold for every 150 additional sugar calories consumed daily, compared with the equivalent amount of calories consumed as fat. And the evidence now suggests that carbs are no better.

Recent research indicates that cutting down on dietary simple carbohydrates is the single most effective approach for reducing all of the features of the metabolic syndrome and should be the primary strategy for treating diabetes, with benefits occurring even in the absence of weight loss.

However, efforts to reduce sugar intake may reduce consumption but may not reduce the prevalence of obesity.
One in four food retailers is now a takeaway accounting for 40% in worst-hit areas.
2/3 adults are overweight in Britain

Not a failure of will-power but the system where the poorest 10% have to spend 75% of their disposable income to afford a healthy diet.

Calorie for calorie unhealthy foods are three times cheaper: Healthy food costs $13.6 per 1000 cals compared with $4.4 per 1000 cals for unhealthy food.

Supermarkets are geared to sell fatty, sugary, salty foods with "healthy"

46% of all food and drink advertising is for confectionery, snacks and soft drink and only 2.5% on fruit and veg.

CHAPTER 21

PORTION CONTROL

THE INCREDIBLE INCREASE IN THE VOLUMES WE EAT

It was not until 1985 that obesity was recognized as a problem by the Center for Disease Control (CDC), the USA Health Authority. In the 1990s Professor Barbara Rowles found that people didn't notice an additional 400 calories added to their food and still ate the same dinner and meals as before.
The latest study found we can eat and extra 1,000 calories but not detect them.

It has been studied and recorded how the Overweight eat larger meals and greatly underestimate calories.

In 1960 David Wallestein, then working for the Balaban Cinema Chain in Chicago realized he could increase profits by doubling the size of the popcorn containers sold at interval. Profits zoomed. He was then head-hunted by McDonald's where its founder, Ray Crock, was reluctant to increase the size of his products but Wallenstein watched as customers tipped up their small carton of chips / fries to slide the salty remnants into their mouths as people didn't want to go back for seconds. And so, super-size cartons were rapidly introduced. Wallestein won and profits zoomed.

Taco Bell then hit on the idea of 'bundling' wherein a starter, main meal, dessert and a drink were offered as a package. This package was then further over-sized so people thought they were getting better value for money. In addition, they would eat even more, the whole servings, as they were presented on a tray and they 'had paid for it'. "I'm going to eat it even if I don't want it" which may be the start of the pervasive 'non-hungry-eating' habit.

Portion size inexorably kept increasing and increasing such that the original 6 1/2 oz (192 ml) coke can now be a 64 oz (1892 ml) 'Double Gulp' which contains 800 calories and 50 teaspoons of sugar. This is a x 10-fold increase!
Restaurants were more successful and profitable if they supersized. Bigger cartons were perceived as better value but cost the restaurant less per profits.

The 20,000 calorie Hamburger

The burger with the most calories in the world can be found at the Heart Attack Grill in Las Vegas, which made national headlines for killing its customers with its over-the-top, gluttonous fare. According to Heart Attack Grill owner Jon Basso, though, death has been good for his restaurant's business. Their 19,900-calorie burger is the Octuple Bypass Burger. The "flatliner fries" are buried and drenched under a greasy layer of mince, and the smallest "bypass burger" is the size of a face. Everything is done in overwhelming sickening excess, and everything is fried in lard - pig fat. People over 350 pounds 'eat for free'.

In the UK Greasy spoon Jesters Diner in Southtown, Great Yarmouth, offers the £15 meal for free to anyone who can finish it in under an hour. Described as a 'heart attack on a plate', the 9lb Kidz Breakfast was so named because it weighs more than an average-sized newborn baby and consists of 12 bacon rashers, 12 sausages, six eggs, four slices of black pudding, four slices of bread and butter, four slices of toast, four slices of fried bread, beans, tomatoes, mushrooms, saute potatoes and an eight-egg cheese and potato omelette - is the calorific equivalent of 12 Big Macs.

Meanwhile on TV we can watch a good-looking young man (for now) overeating obscene amounts in 'Man versus Food'. All this may sound a bit of not-every-day fun, but these people have got it wrong. Their cost to the nation's health bill will be incredible and only amortized by their premature deaths.

Like binge drinking it starts as an exception, a bit of fun, becomes accepted, then pervasive and, as for super-sizing, finally regarded as the norm.

Based on the Coke size all, or *most, of our food portions are now 10 times more than the original size.* Larger carton size is perceived as 'better value'.

Before portions were deliberately increased obesity rates were only 1 in 10 in the UK but have increased to 1:4 and 1:3 in the USA. This is officially an epidemic. The UK Government commissioned medical reports, but these were buried and never published because the Fast Food Lobby spent some $100 million to oppose them. The Fast Food Industry claimed that it was 'reduced activity' by the younger generation which led to the increasing rate of obesity but one such report found that there had been no reduction in activity – just an increase in portion size and calorie-dense, nutrient-poor processed foods. Advertising Agencies of the Fast Food Industry then targeted Mothers to include fudge / fat sticks in their kids' lunch boxes.

Eating out became cheaper and faster. By offering fast service many more people could be processed. A 15 second per person speed up amounted to a 1% increase in profit or $500 million pa in the UK. Eating in public became acceptable.

Unlike the Okinawans who always leave something on the plate and stop eating before they feel full and who are among the longest living and leanest people on earth, we now eat until we are not just full, but stuffed. If we consistently overeat, we 'stretch' the stomach (reset the pressor-receptors) such that unless we get this new larger volume, we feel hungry. We are now consuming more Calories than we need. We are getting fatter.

Bags of crisps got bigger and bigger, but people didn't reduce the size of their meals despite eating all the crisps. Between 1996 and 2013 researchers analyzed the calorie, sodium, saturated fat and trans-fat content of popular menu items served at three national fast-food US chains. They found that average calories, sodium, and saturated fat stayed relatively constant, albeit at high levels. Among the three USA chains, calories in a large cheeseburger meal, with fries and a regular cola beverage, ranged from 1144 to 1757 over the years and among restaurants, representing 57% to 88% of the approximately 2000 calories most people should eat per day.

People have or used to have set volume intakes but then, if the volume stays the same, but the calorie content is increased (by eating hi-calorie junk), then fat is put on. If then the intake default volume size is reset (up) there is even greater gain.

We all had a smaller default volume size when we were slim but by chronically overeating this default volume is now greater: We 'have' to eat more food to feel full. If you are to lose weight you must eat less, either volume or calories and in practical terms this means volume.

The Pima Indians

The most classic example that obesity is caused by overeating and eating the wrong foods is best demonstrated by the Pima Indians, who some many years ago were separated into two groups, (I seem to remember it was due to the Colorado River flooding, but I can't find any reference to this).

Half the tribe stayed in the USA while the other half were forcibly separated and relocated to Mexico. Those remaining in the USA, the American Arizona Pima Indians, currently have the highest rates of diabetes and obesity in the United States. That wasn't always the case. They were lean until around 1890 when their water supply was overtaken by American settlers upstream. The United States government then began subsidizing the tribe's food -- much of it containing sugar and white flour, and obesity and diabetes rates soared.

By distinct contrast the contingent of Pima who relocated to the Sierra Madre mountains of Mexico continued traditional farming, and the vast majority of Mexico's Pima Indians have maintained healthy weights.

Those left in America with access to cars, processed and deep-fried foods now have the highest rates of obesity, diabetes 2, renal disease and premature deaths while their genetically identical cohorts in Mexico walk 2 miles to school, hand grind corn for tortillas and plough the fields, don't have any obesity and little diabetes, heart or kidney disease.

PIMA INDIANS	USA	MEXICO
Diabetes	34.2 – 40.8%	5.6 – 8.5%
Weight	215 pounds	145 pounds
Physical work	3.1 hours	22 hours
Fiber	12 – 15 g/day	50g / day

It would only seem common sense that this same tribe shared the same gut biome, unless the differences in their diet also altered their gut microbes but, be that as it may, the most obvious difference is the change from a primitive, fresh food diet to one of processed foods, deep frying and reduced exercise.

Epidemic of Obesity and Overweight linked to increased food supply
A WHO study investigated the associations between changes in national food supply and average population body weight in 24 high, 27 middle and 18 low-income countries. Both body weight and food energy supply had increased in 81% of the 69 countries between 1971 and 2010. It was found that the increases in food supply explained the increases in average population weight.

Between 1980 and 2013, the proportion of adults globally who were overweight -- i.e. those with a BMI of 25 kg/m2 or more -- increased from 28.8% to 36.9% in men, and from 29.8% to 38% in women. A person with a BMI of 30 or more is considered obese.

Percent of adults who are overweight or obese:

USA:	=	69.0%
UK:	=	67.0% of men and 57.0% of women
Australia:	=	70.3% of men and 55.7% of women

WHO Study of 69 countries found: Between 1971 and 2008:
  USA food intake increased by 768 calories a day
  Canada food intake increased by 559 calories per person per day
  Fiji food intake increased by 550 calories per day

In 1960 World Food Energy Consumption was 2250 cals /person / day.
In 2004 it was 2760 cals. This is a daily increase of over 500 calories a day when just 20 are needed to gain weight and 100 to become obese.

Fast Food Industry 'Sweeteners"
The Fast Food Industry is trying, alarmingly successfully, to blame lack of exercise rather than sugar as the cause of the obesity epidemic (as alluded to before). They have nobbled Parliamentary Reports in the UK and in the USA as Cardiologist, Larry Husten, wrote in his CardioBrief 25th September 2015:
'Large food and beverage companies have been insinuating their way into the healthcare discussion for many years... the newly elected president of the Institute of Medicine, cardiologist Victor Dzau, was a member of the Pepsico Board of Directors. In 2012 the president of the American College of Cardiology was chosen by the Coca-Cola Company to carry the Olympic Flame. (Steven Blair, another co-author of the *JACC* paper, was also *chosen by Coke to be a*

torch-bearer.) Coke also pays a lot of money to the National Heart Lung and Blood Institute to put a red dress logo on the Diet Coke label, while the American Heart Association has struck deals with, among others, Cheetos and Subway... a review of systematic reviews examining the association between sugar-sweetened beverages and weight gain and obesity... the papers in which the authors reported no conflict of interest, 10 out of the 12 findings supported the association between sugar-sweetened beverages and weight gain or obesity. In stark contrast, 5 out of the 6 papers with industry support failed to find evidence for any such association. In other words, systematic reviews with industry support were 5 times more likely to find no significant association'.

Almost all food, beverage products marketed by music stars are unhealthy. Sugary drinks, fast food and sweets are among the most common products and advertising these is contributing to the great rise in childhood and teen obesity.

Sugar Beverages
Soft drink, fruit punches contain large amounts of readily absorbable sugars and are associated with a greater magnitude of weight gain and an increased risk for development of type 2 diabetes.

On any given day, half the people in the U.S. consume sugary drinks; 1 in 4 get at least 200 calories from such drinks; and 5% get at least 567 calories—equivalent to four cans of soda.

Sugary drinks (soda, energy, sports drinks) are the top calorie source in teens' diets (226 calories per day), beating out pizza (213 calories / day).

Many people wrongly believe that obesity is entirely due to lack of exercise, a perception, as noted, that is firmly rooted in corporate marketing. But it is the excess sugar and refined-simple carbs, not physical inactivity, which are behind the surge in obesity. Regular exercise is a key to staving off serious disease, such as diabetes and heart disease but our calorie laden diets now generate more ill health than physical inactivity, alcohol, and smoking combined.

The public relations tactics of the food industry are "chillingly similar to those of Big Tobacco," which deployed denial, doubt, confusion and "bent scientists" to convince the public that smoking was not linked to lung cancer and used Celebrity endorsements of sugary drinks and the association of junk food and sport.

Sugar calories promote fat storage and hunger. Fat calories induce fullness or satiation. The prevalence of diabetes increases 11-fold for every 150 additional sugar calories consumed daily, compared with the equivalent amount of calories consumed as fat. Other refined carbs are no better.

Oversized meals have been shown to be a factor in obesity[67]
94% of the most popular main dishes served in sit-down restaurants in Brazil, China, Finland, Ghana and India and 72% of those purchased over the counter from fast food outlets contained more than 600 kilocalories (kcal), the benchmark recently recommended by the United Kingdom's National Health Service (NHS) to help reduce the global obesity epidemic.

SUPER-SIZE ME

Ronald McDonald
The original Ronald McDonald ate so many Big-Macs he became obese and they sacked him.

Obesity: The New Phenomenon
While obesity has been known for centuries, such generalized incidence of epidemic proportions, is a recent phenomenon only recognized medically since 1985 and formally recognized as a global epidemic in1997 by the World Health Organization (WHO).
If you think about it, if processed foods were slowly introduced after WW2 and were to have an effect, it would be first noticed when these people were in their 30s. 1950 + 35 years = 1985 when Obesity, not just overweight, was first recognized. A coincidence? I think not.

To Gain 269% Weight:
As in the Nutrition Chapter, in the early 1970s a study on obesity was done with an all-you-can-eat "Supermarket Diet" that incorporated milk chocolate, chocolate-chip cookies and marshmallows and they gained 269% (compared with those on a normal diet). OK it was done on rats, but the message is clear...you can do it too![68]

---

[67] *British Medical Journal, 30 Jan 2019*
[68] Sclafani, A., & Springer, D. (1976). Dietary obesity in adult rats: Similarities to hypothalamic and human obesity syndromes. *Physiology & Behavior, 17*, 461-471

Wider Seats, Reinforced Operating Tables

The number of Americans who are too grossly overweight to fit into an airline seats has increased by 350% in 30 years. Operating tables now have to be made stronger to take the weight of the fatter population. This is also the case for most Western societies.

Over the past 33 years, overweight and obesity rates among adults have increased by 27.5% and the 'Diseases of Affluence', heart disease, strokes, blood pressure, hyperlipidaemia, diabetes, cancer of the colon and their downstream cousins of arthritis and depression, are our greatest killers. Or, to be more accurate, the cause of our *premature* disabilities or deaths. Most of us are headed for a Nursing Home or dying before we should. The latest USA report provided a detailed assessment of changes over time in fast-food menu offerings over 30 years, from 1986 to 2016. Portion sizes increased significantly, and the energy (kilocalories) and sodium increased significantly.[69]

The Portion Size Effect

The portion size effect is the tendency of people to eat more when larger portions are served.

When served larger portions of typical meals or snacks, children, between the ages of three and five, consumed more food over time, both by weight and calories and did not self-regulate to control this increase.[70]

---

[69] Journal of the Academy of Dietetics and Nutrition
DOI: https://doi.org/10.1016/j.jand.2018.12.004
[70] American Journal of Clinical Nutrition 2019

CHAPTER 22

The PERFECT STORM

Causes of this Overweight-Obesity Epidemic: Not the Perfect Storm but The Perfect Hurricane

- New processed foods our bodies can't metabolize
- New synthetic, often untested, additives
- The chemical industry makes these foods delicious, mouth-watering, irresistible by achieving the Industry "bliss point"
- Commercial Fast Food Industry whose budget exceeds that of most Governments who fund Political Parties and have infiltrated Health Authorities
- Refining of natural foods: 95% fiber is lost & other nutrients
- Increased salt & sugar to commercial foods altering our tastes
- Increased affluence
- Availability, affordability and convenience of such foods
- Fast foods three times cheaper than healthy foods
- The poor environmentally and economically conditioned to prefer fast food
- Reduced fresh foods especially fruit and vegetables
- Prepared meals cheaper, easier faster (and often better tasting) than cooking and more convenient
- Rows of drive in Fast Food outlets – miss one, no problem drive into the next or the next…
- Unrelenting advertising, hoardings and logos
- TV ads for high sugar sweets specifically aimed at children
- Fast unhealthy food is three times cheaper than healthy foods
- Supermarkets push unhealthy foods
- Rows of dazzling packaged foods and sweets in Supermarkets
- Fast Food Industry pays for supermarket displays, promotions
- Fast food available 24 hrs a day seven days a week
- Increased portion sizes and consequent expectations
- Increased leisure
- Increased affluence to afford sugar drinks and alcohol
- Increased labor-saving devices, less physical work

- Increased sedentary behaviors, less activities
- Decreased exercise
- Women in workforce: No "little wife" home preparing meals
- Increased modern day pressures and stresses
- Long work days. Don't feel like cooking when we get home
- Most people live in towns or cities – no vegetable gardens
- Claims for unproven health benefits allowed by Governments
- 4,000 calories per day of food produced for every person on the planet. We need only 1,500 to 2,000 cals
- We cannot appreciate eating 1,000 calories more a day
- We only need 20cals a day to put on weight, 100cals a day to become obese
- Americans are eating 778cals a day more
- We are eating too much, for too long, insidiously every day without realizing it and it's the wrong food

All these evolved together at the same time, since WW2, and they have combined to add to each other multiplying the total effect. They have also been insidious such that we don't even notice them but take all for granted whereas "Grandma wouldn't recognize them'.

Most of us could not conceive chopping wood to get hot water, having a vegetable garden and chooks, let alone killing, gutting and plucking them, walking to the shop and lugging home the shopping, walking to school or long distances every day to the public transport. Money was tight and food often not plentiful or affordable. Yet this was normal living just a generation ago, when people were not overweight.

Now we hop in our cars, park immediately outside the supermarket or even drive thru to get pre-prepared meals or pizzas delivered, don't have vegetable gardens to dig let alone eat fresh produce and we have the money to buy these delicious, unnatural junk foods in excess. And it is worse for the poor who have no idea of nutrition and prefer junk, take-away with shops in their neighborhood catering for this processed junk.

There is no mystery why we are the fattest generation in the history of the world and, if you want to really lose weight, you have to get back to this more natural lifestyle.

I

HEALTH

CHAPTER 23

HEALTH

THE BENEFITS of WEIGHT CONTROL

Risks Even If Fit
People who are overweight or obese by BMI criteria, even lacking several well-established cardiometabolic risk factors, are at significantly increased risk of coronary heart disease (CHD), cerebrovascular disease, and heart failure compared with normal-weight people without those risk factors, concludes a study using a massive UK 3.5 million adults primary-care database.[71]

Calorie Restriction Increases Longevity
Previous studies over the past 85 years have supported the notion that calorie restriction can increase lifespan by reducing inflammation and other chronic disease risk factors. Chronic inflammation has been shown to create successions of destructive reactions that damage cells, thus playing a major role in the development of age-related diseases such as cancer, heart disease, and dementia. According to the Centers for Disease Control and Prevention (CDC), seven of the top 10 causes of death in 2010 were chronic diseases, with heart disease and cancer accounting for nearly 48 percent of all deaths.
A recent study examined these effects over two years on healthy, normal or slightly over- weight individuals and found that caloric restriction reduces inflammation without compromising other key functions of the immune system. The test group had a significant and persistent reduction in inflammatory markers
It is considered that it is certainly feasible for the average person to maintain a 10-15 percent calorie restriction as a strategy for long-term health benefit.

Estimated Benefits of 10% Weight Loss
- o *BP*: Fall of 10 mm in systolic and diastolic blood pressure in hypertense patients
- o *Diabetes*
    - o Fall of up to 50% in fasting glucose in newly diagnosed patients.
    - o 3 to 4yr increased life span

---

[71] September 11, 2017 in the *Journal of the American College of Cardiology.*

- *People at Risk of Diabetes*
  - 30% fall in fasting insulins
  - 30% increase in insulin sensitivity
  - 40% - 60% fall in incidence of diabetes
- *Lipids*
  - Fall 10% in total cholesterol
  - Fall 15% in LDL (bad) cholesterol
  - Fall 30% in triglycerides
  - Rise 8% in HDL (good) cholesterol
- *Mortality*
  - 20% fall in all-cause mortality
  - 30% fall in deaths related to diabetes
  - 40% fall in deaths related to obesity

CONSEQUENCES OF OVERWEIGHT / OBESITY

Medical

Diabetes 2

Metabolic Syndrome

CardioVascular: Hypertension, heart attacks, Coronary Heart Disease, heart Failure, atrial fibrillation, strokes, Varicose veins, piles, Dyslipidaemia (cholesterol / triglycerides)

Cancer

Breathlessness, fatigue, lassitude, aches, pains, indigestion, heat intolerance

Sleep Apnoea, snoring, somnolence, poor concentration

Gallstones, Gall Bladder Disease, Cirrhosis

Increased morbidity and mortality – all causes

Osteoarthritis, neck problems / spondylosis – facet locking, Low back pain

Hyperuricaemia and gout

Pregnancy Complications, Foetal defects, Impaired fertility / Polycystic ovary syndrome, menstrual disorders

Impotence

Hirsutism

Anesthetic risk

Depression, low self-esteem, lowered confidence, personality changes

Excess sweat, rashes, intertrigo, thrush, chafing, hygiene problems

Neglected feet

Social

Psychological

Social Penalties

Discrimination – less likely to be hired or promoted

Obese employees have twice the rate of absenteeism & compensation claims

For every 1 kg excess employees are paid $500 p.a. less

Social derision; the butt of jokes

Embarrassment with seating, crowds

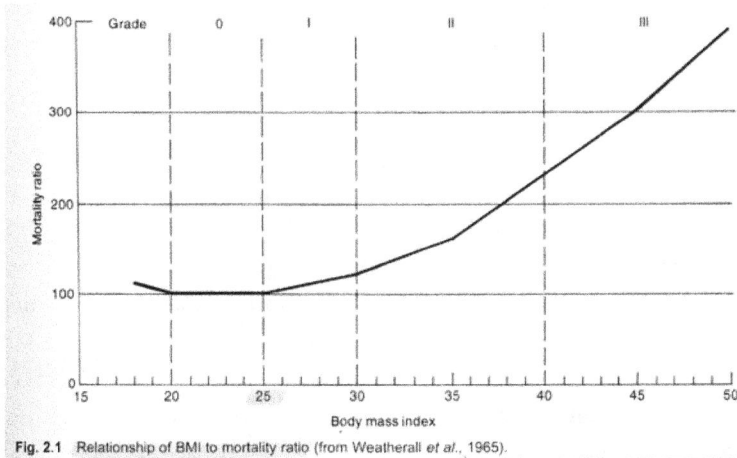

Fig. 2.1 Relationship of BMI to mortality ratio (from Weatherall et al., 1965).

Never Healthier

It has been documented that the British were never healthier than in WW2 when food was restricted, and exercise increased as mimicked in the following Cuban experience. During the economic crisis in Cuba (1991–1995), food and gas shortages resulted in lower food intake, greater energy expenditure (e.g., through walking and bicycling as alternatives to motorized transport), and weight loss across the population. Since then, the Cuban economy has recovered, and Cubans are less active and have gained weight. During the economic crisis, daily per capita energy intake was 2400 kcal, and 80% of adults were physically active; average weight loss during 5 years was 5.5 kg. During the economic recovery period (1996–2010), daily energy intake rose to 3200 kcal, the proportion of overweight and obese adults increased 20%, and the proportion of physically active adults fell to 55%. Between 1997 and 2009, diabetes incidence and prevalence doubled. During the "weight rebound phase" (2002–2009), diabetes-related mortality increased, and previously declining cardiovascular and overall mortality returned to pre-1991 rates.

Waist Not Want Not

Abdominal obesity independently predicts mortality risk.

Every ten-centimeter increase in waist circumference was linked to a 29 per cent higher risk of heart failure.

For example, men with a waist circumference of 105 cm virtually doubled their risk of heart failure compared with men whose waist measured 83 cm. For women, the risk was 80 per cent higher with a waist circumference of 90 cm than with a waist circumference of 70 cm.

Medical Aim

The medical aim in losing weight and getting fit is *to reduce Intra-abdominal or Visceral fat*, which is laid down with increasing overweight and then surrounds our abdominal organs. The problem is that this Visceral Fat now starts producing oestrogen in both women and men. This may help reduce the hot flushes in women but is far worse overall. In men it effectively performs a therapeutic gelding. This oestrogen signals the testes not to produce testosterone and so yet more fat is laid down and eventually the man develops breasts, then neck fat which makes him snore at night and cuts off the oxygen to his pituitary causing it to further signal the testes to produce yet less testosterone.

The 'man' now gets fatter, afternoon fatigue and naps set in. He now needs Viagra and develops insulin resistance, diabetes ii, blood pressure, dyslipidaemias and dies prematurely from all causes. Women's risks, however, as stated, are worse if they gain waist fat.

If you exercise, while you may not lose weight you do lose fat, replacing it with muscle. And the fat you lose is the deleterious intra-abdominal fat. Just aim to lose 5% to 10%, hopefully 15%.

If you are a male, get your waist below 102 cm and if you are a women get it below 88 cm and both BMIs at 25 (if possible).

Visceral fat

VAT = Visceral Adipose Tissue per sq cm or Intraabdominal fat or the fat that is actually *inside your abdomen* and not just that hanging over the belt. Visceral fat is deep and accumulates around abdominal organs and is associated with metabolic problems / syndrome.

It is the worst because it produces oestrogen the female hormone which gives the male little feminized breasts as well as feeding back to further reduce testosterone production. Measurement is usually by sophisticated x-ray/CT techniques wherein a teenage girl has about 60 VAT (in the days when they were not obese). Adults should have a reading < 110 and certainly < 130. Between 110 and 130 exponential metabolic problems occur and increase eg oestrogen production and insulin resistance. Men have X2 % VAT compared with premenopausal women. Neck fat is proportionate to VAT, hence Sleep Apnoea reflects VAT.

TOFI: Thin Outside Fat Inside

It is possible and reasonably frequent that a person can look to not be overweight but have excess visceral fat. An MRI is the only way to confirm this. Many 'coat-hanger' models suffer from this. They starve themselves like anorexics to be thin but don't do any real exercise and their muscles have wasted.

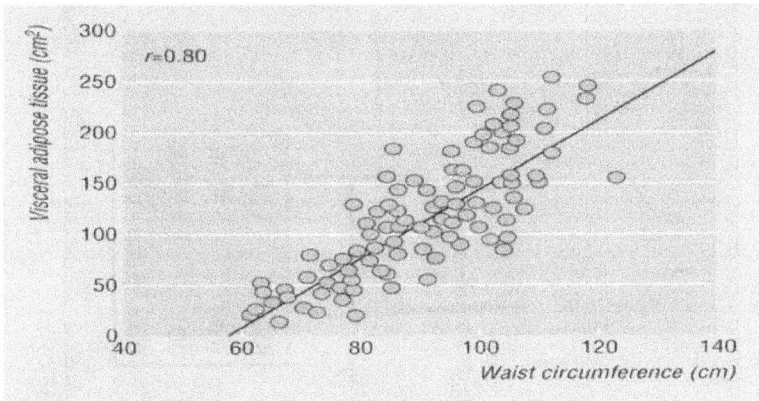

Arch Int Med 2007;167:886-92

Danger Signs: Neck fat, increasing breast tissue, the afternoon nap.

VAT, independent of obesity, is a major determinant of insulin resistance, dyslipidaemia and the Metabolic Syndrome. Insulin Resistance is directly related to VAT.

VAT volume is relatively small: 20% of total fat in obese men and 6% of total fat in obese women

VAT exposes the liver to high levels of Free Fatty Acids and Glycerol (fats), increasing hepatic Glucose and Triglyceride production and decreases Insulin clearance and raised insulin sensitivity to increase the risk of Cardiovascular Disease.

Age reduces Growth Hormone as does the rise in VAT which perpetuates central obesity. Best to lose the fat by eating less and exercising more and so reverse this vicious cycle. Moderate exercise _brisk_ walking 30 min a day / 3 hr a week halts accumulation of VAT

* 45 min / day 5 days / week reduced it 3.4 to 6.9% pa while maintaining same calorie intake as before

* High intensity (jogging 3hr/20 miles/wk) reduced it by 7% pa

* Remaining sedentary gained 9% visceral fat in 6/12. A CT Scan to measure this VAT is not absolutely necessary - all you need is an abdomen < 102 cm if male and <88cm if female at the waist (irrespective of height).

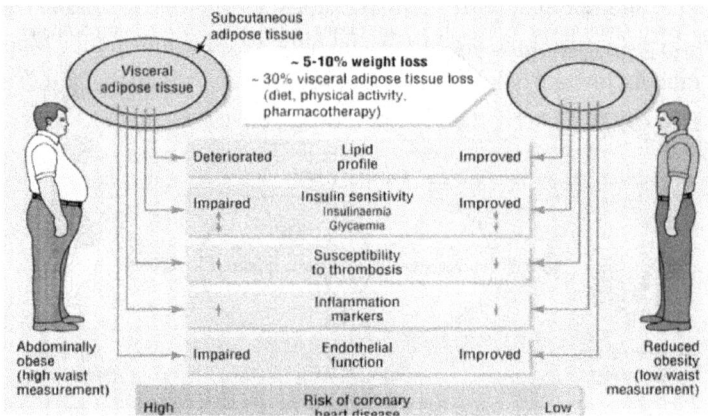

The Metabolic Syndrome: is the constellation of

1)Obesity

2) diabetes

3) hypertension

4) hypertriglygeridaemia.

The increase in mortality for each additional unit increase is:

For men: 1) 64%, 2) 95%, 3) 152% 4) 295%

For women it is much worse: 1) 343%, 2)403%, 3) 532% 4) 1239%

It gets much worse for women if their waist exceeds 95 cm.

Abdominal Obesity – The Consequences

The Metabolic Syndrome: Increasing BMI : 4 Major Problems

1.)Hyperinsulinaemia - insulin resistance

2). Hyperglycaemia - diabetes

3). Hyperlipidaemia

4). Hypertension

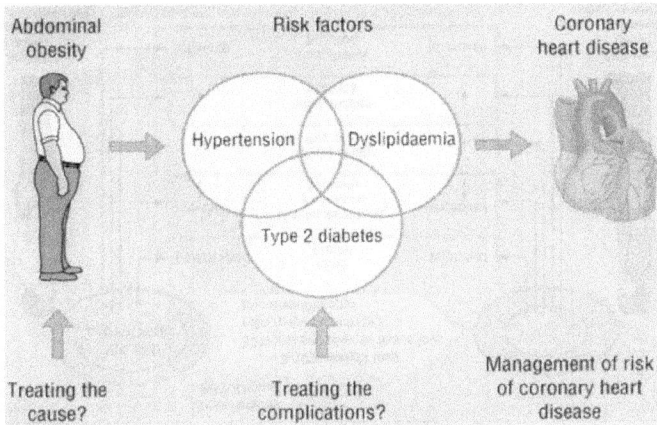

Research indicates that cutting down on dietary simple /refined carbohydrates is the single most effective approach for reducing all of the features of the metabolic syndrome and should be the primary strategy for treating diabetes, with benefits occurring even in the absence of weight loss.

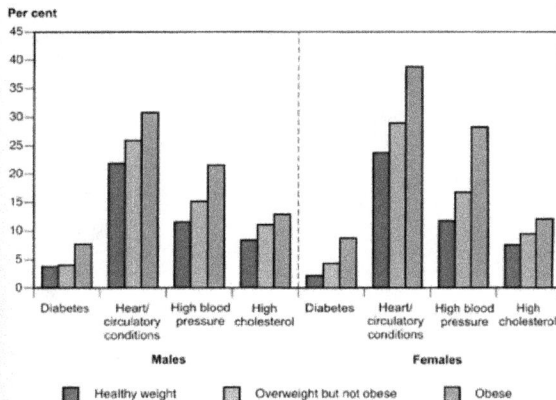

Notes

1. Age-standardised to the 2001 Australian population.

2. Diabetes, high blood pressure and high blood cholesterol results for persons aged 25 years and over. Heart/ circulatory conditions for persons aged 20 years and over.

3. Based on self-reported data.

Source: AIHW analysis of the 2001 National Health Survey.

Figure 3.4: Proportion of adults with selected conditions by BMI category, 2001

J

HISTORY

OBESITY
DIETS

CHAPTER 24

THE HISTORY OF OBESITY

Obesity was known in Roman times. At age 55 Henry Vlll was believed to weigh more than 320 pounds (not enough to get a free meal at the Heart Attack Restaurant in America at 350 pounds), ate 5000 calories a day and 70 pints of ale a week. Obesity was then the fashion vogue. Lord Byron, as well as being 'mad, bad and dangerous to know' and like Henry V111 a fabulous athlete when young, fought obesity all his life. Fat and prosperous was the cliché as only the rich could afford excess food and leisure. Now it is the urban or small-town poor who are fat. In the absence of photography and medical measurements we can only look at the art of the times. The first sculpture known is 'The Earth Mother' Venus of Willendorf of 24,000–22,000 BC whose fatness many feel represent fertility but was obesity common? Greek and Roman art idealized the athlete and the golden mean and there are no fat statues and until the renaissance only the low socioeconomic status were depicted as obese. During the Renaissance some of the upper class began flaunting their large size, as can be seen in portraits of Henry VIII of England and Alessandro del Borro. Rubens (1577–1640) regularly depicted full-bodied women in his pictures. These Rubenesque women, however, still maintained the "hourglass" shape. During the 19th century, views on obesity changed in the Western world. After centuries of obesity being synonymous with wealth and social status, slimness began to be seen as

The desirable standard.

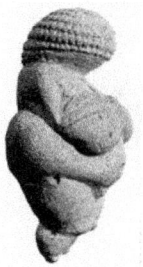

Venus of Willendorf

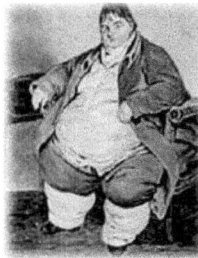

Daniel Lambert, Britain's
fattest man 1806 >50st (700lb or 318kg)

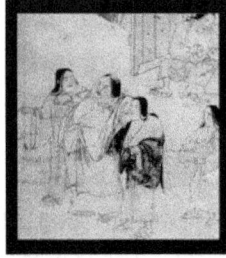

In medieval Japan C12 obesity was considered to be found in the rich as portrayed in this scroll of a money-lender. Perhaps this was a case of 'fat and prosperous' – gaining weight in direct proportion to her increasing income and therefore ability to buy more food and, of course, her increased weight made her more sedentary. At that stage she may well have been able to shed some weight, but best achieved at the same rate she put it on. Instead, we take years to insidiously put it on but want it off immediately – hence the 'success' of the fad diets. During the Middle Ages and the Renaissance obesity was often seen as a sign of wealth, and was relatively common among the elite.

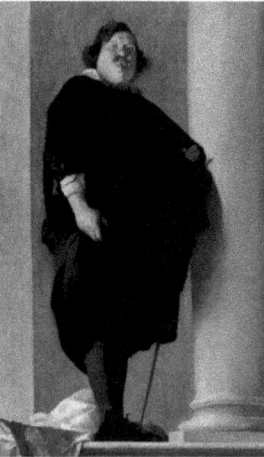

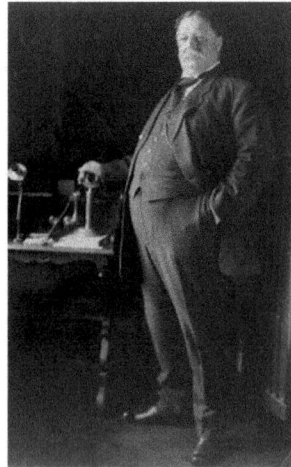

Tuscan General Alessandro del Borro, 1645

United States President William Howard Taft 1908

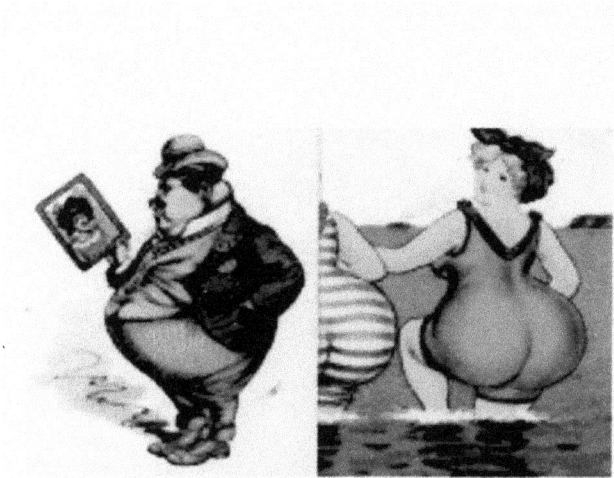

Apple and Pear

Men are apple shaped which is more metabolically harmful (waist). Women are Pear shaped which is metabolically protective (hips) but worse than for men if they gain waist fat. However, making obesity an object of humor has impeded understanding the medical consequences.

Severe or morbid obesity

Severe or morbid obesity is a profound medical problem which has now been classified as a disease. As such it is not addressed here.

CHAPTER 25

HISTORY OF DIETS

SCAMS and FADS

What has this got to do with you now wanting to lose weight?
Well, the point is to wean you off all these Fads and Scams. But if you don't know
they are scams you may be tempted to try and try and try them.

There have been, arguably, more scams and books on weight losing diets than on
any other health subject.

Be that as it may, ALL diets, fad diets, commercial weight clinics programs and
plans purely depend on smoke and mirrors to fool you into eating less.

Sad but true.

Why other diets don't work is because most, if not all, diet-weight loss books are
dishonest or deluded.

The best of them may realize this but nevertheless promote their system in the
attempt to help you lose weight.

Some have elements and vestiges of truth but not the whole, honest truth.

Some are deluded and actually believe their plans with all the fervor of the Zealot.

Most are just money-making scams.

Basically, there is or are no diet(s) that will work for everyone. You have to do is
find one, or a system, that works for you. The best have been detailed.

Here are 2,619 years of diets which keep being repeated and resurrected.

Why?

Because they didn't work to begin with.
Individually they overwhelm us and become the latest craze or Fad Diet. My wife

and I have sensible friends who are forever on one or another (but they don't lose weight). These Fads depend on didactic regimes and lay out strict menus under the guise of 'low-carbs' or 'balancing the acid-alkali' or some other rubbish when *all* they are doing is getting you to eat less than 1,200 to 1,500 calories a day and using their pseudo-science as a gimmick to entrap you.

"The problem with common sense is that it is not very common" as Churchill observed, but use your common sense to glance through this history to see how, indeed, 'history repeats itself' and how, if the lo-carb, hi-protein smoke and mirrors are withdrawn, they are all scams to reduce your intake and have been being peddled and re-presented to new gullible generation after generation (the Cabbage Soup diet has grabbed every generation since 300AD!).

That is why they don't work long-term and why the **Slim 4 Life** is a totally unique **Program**, not just a diet, which approaches weight reduction from a completely different aspect and direction, now offers you the best plan and from my 50 years of clinical medicine the *only* plan.

Fasting Diets, which unlike most are to be commended, are as old as 'God's dog'. Daniel, in the Old Testament semi-fasted for 10 or 21 days, no booze, plenty of veg (sounds familiar) and felt great afterwards. I mean, at the outset they are at least honest (and effective) because they insist you eat less and not con you to eat some cabbage, raw-food, hi-fat, different ratios of protein, carbs and fat, the bottom of the cockatoo's cage, chew your food 1100 times and what-have-you, or any other ridiculous gimmick they can think up.

The Daniel Fast is drawn from the Book of Daniel, which appears in the Old Testament. Daniel decides to avoid the rich, indulgent foods that surround him and have *"nothing but vegetables to eat and water to drink"* for 10 days. (Some translations interpret vegetables as pulses, meaning foods grown from seeds.) A later reference says, *"I, Daniel, mourned for three weeks. I ate no choice food; no meat or wine touched my lips; and I used no lotions at all until the three weeks were over."* At the end of the fast, he was healthy.

According to scholars the Book of Daniel gives clear internal dates such as *"the third year of the reign of king Jehoiakim,"* (1:1), which is 606 BC.
Research by the University of Memphis found that the Daniel Diet after just three

weeks, can begin to lower risk factors for metabolic and cardiovascular disease, such as high blood pressure and cholesterol, and reduce oxidative stress. Maybe he was also healthy before his fast, but he sure was thinner – an estimated 6 pounds or 2.7 kg from duplicate studies.

The Keto Diet: Using starvation to treat seizures can be found in the Bible and in references as far back to 500 B.C. In 1911, two physicians in Paris tried starving 20 persons and found that seizures improved. In 1921, the Ketogenic diet was evolved as a long-term treatment for epilepsy without actual starvation. With the development of modern epilepsy drugs, the Keto Diet lapsed only to now be revived.

Fad diets, the current short-term craze, are usually with little or pseudo-scientific basis, but advertising extravagant claims. They are generally restrictive, obsessive and unsustainable.

The first commercial or wide-spread fad diet programs began popping up in the 19th century in America, in the late 1820s with the Sylvester Graham's Diet, considered the first "Fad diet". Thereafter sanitarium health spas such as that of Dr Kellog of Corn Flake and anti-masturbation fame, but before then there were odd diets which, had there been the mass media, would have been fads then as some have been re-discovered to be come modern day fads. For example, low carb diets date back to 1825.

In the 6th century BC Olympic athletes followed specific fads such as favoring cheese, figs and grains but avoiding pork, fish and beans. It is claimed that the famous Olympic wrestler Milo of Kroton of this era would consume up to 40lb (18kg) of meat and bread in one sitting. He was obviously not 'dieting'!

Originally, the Greek word "diatia" meant a sensible, moderate and dutiful *way of living* with no specific reference to food. Later it came to be associated with foods associated with that lifestyle and while it is still used in that context, it has now evolved, and is most commonly used, to describe an eating regime to lose weight.

The 'Father of Medicine' the Greek physician Hippocrates in the 3rd century BC, recommended a diet of light and emollient foods, slow running, hard work, wrestling, sea-water enemas, walking about naked and vomiting after lunch. The Greeks believed that being fat was morally and physically detrimental, the result of luxury and corruption, so food and living should be plain with nothing to unduly stir the passions or arouse the appetites. This was the first documented diet or "diatia".

The following, I assure you, are just the highlights of a very big, obese Iceberg of silly diets. Today, as you read this, there will be over 100 such Fad diets inviting you to fail.

2,600BC The Daniel Diet

500BC The Keto Diet

500BC: Olympic Athlete Fad Diets

175BC: The Cabbage and Urine Diet
Cato the Elder was a Roman statesman, writer and public speaker who was a massive fan of cabbage; he not only promoted eating plenty of cabbage but also drinking the urine of people who had a diet high in cabbage. It is reported that Cato continued to believe in the power of cabbage even after this diet "failed to save the lives of his wife and son". It had a big resurgence in the 1950s and even today some advocates still urge cabbage soup diets.

300AD: John Chrysostom claimed fasting promotes health

1087: dieting does not seem to have been recorded between and 1087 when it was mentioned how William the Conqueror had become too heavy to ride his horse, so he decided that he would stop eating solid foods and only partake in a "liquid diet" that consisted only of alcohol in an attempt to lose weight. It must have worked as he later died from a fall off his horse but was still too big for the casket. This may be the first recorded instance in which an individual changed his or her food intake habits to lose weight.

1820: Lord Byron (the poet): The Vinegar Diet.
The Vinegar Diet (yes it's back too) of potatoes flattened and drenched in apple vinegar or drinking water mixed with apple cider vinegar. It also caused vomiting and diarrhea. But he also purged himself and wore heavy clothing all day to cause sweating.

1825: Physiologie du goût (The Physiology of Taste): Lo-Carbs
French lawyer and physician Jean-Anthelme Brillat-Savarin's pioneered the low-carb diet observing *"Tell me what you eat, and I will tell you what you are."*

1820s late: Sylvester Graham's Diet:
Considered the first "Fad diet", Graham was a Presbyterian Minister who combined his strict religious beliefs and temperance proposing a plain vegetarian diet to prevent the "over-stimulation" of other foods which caused "immoral behavior, gluttony and promiscuity". He invented the cracker and had a huge following including John Harvey Kellogg (see later). He claimed his diet would prolong life to 100 years but died aged 57.

1830: Tapeworms
Victorians and 1920s Hollywood:

1863: Lo-Carb Diet. William Banting was a notable English undertaker.
Formerly obese, he was advised to lose weight by his doctor and to begin journaling about his "diet" i.e. keep a diet diary. His diet was worked out by Dr William Harvey but Banting, while acknowledging this, privately published 'his' diet and became the first to popularise a weight loss diet based on limiting the intake of carbohydrates, especially those of a starchy or sugary nature. Just as did Brillat-Savarin, and now popular again.

1880 High fat, low carb diet Germany. Popularized again by Dr Atkins 1972

1885 No breakfast and Raw Food faddists. Raw food is making a comeback

Late 1800s: Arsenic Diet Pills
These Victorian diet pills were advertised as "miracle cures" which could "speed up the metabolism". Although the amount of arsenic within the pills was small, these were still very dangerous and posed the risk of arsenic poisoning; especially when the pills were taken in high doses. It also didn't help matters that the labels of these pills didn't always declare that they contained arsenic[5]!

Early 1900s: The Tapeworm Diet
This was first recorded (as above) in 1830, reputedly reached maximum vogue in the Hollywood of the 1920s and last recorded when the opera singer Maria Callas, the paramour of Aristotle Onassis, see below. People would voluntarily ingest tapeworms in order to decrease nutrient absorption and promote vomiting and diarrhea to achieve weight loss. This has multiple risks associated with it such as: organ swelling, anaphylaxis, infections of the digestive system, appendicitis, damaged vision, meningitis, epilepsy, dementia or even death in severe cases. It doesn't seem quite worth the risk to drop a few pounds…

1895-1919: Fletcherism Diet "Chew and spit".
Fletcher, 'The Great Masticator', was an ex-whaler, pirate, sharp-shooter, opera manager, businessman (art dealer) and self-taught nutritionist who became the 20th century's first diet guru with John D. Rockefeller, Franz Kafka and Henry James as adherents. Chewing food thoroughly until liquid (32 to 100 to 700 times) and then spitting it out was the idea behind the Fletcherism Diet. Fletcherites were also urged to eat only when they were really, really hungry and to never eat when their emotions were running high.
Not bad advice really and a small 2011 study showed that higher chewing counts reduced food intake.[72]

1903: President William Howard Taft pledges to slim down after getting stuck in the White House bathtub.
He apparently then kept a daily log and adopted a low-calorie, low-fat diet.

1911: Hereward Carrington 'The Fasting Cure"
Carrington embraced different food fads and experimented with fasting, fruitarianism and raw food diets. His book *Vitality, Fasting and Nutrition* is over six hundred pages and was negatively reviewed in the British Medical Journal. He died aged 78.
1911, two physicians in Paris tried starving 20 persons and found that seizures improved. In **1921**, the Ketogenic diet was evolved as a long-term treatment for epilepsy without actual starvation.

---

[72] Appetite 2011;57:295-298

1917 Dr. Lulu Hunt Peters published *Diet and Health*
She introduced the concept of counting calories and so new was the concept she even included how to pronounce it. It sold more than two million copies and became the first bestselling American diet book. Dr. Peters urged readers to view the calorie as a measurement and rather than judge meals by portion size. It was recommended that the amount of calories in any given food were counted and totaled each day. She concluded that to lose weight it was important to stay under 1,200 calories a day.
Authors Note: She was correct! But portions have now also increased at least 10fold.
It has been observed that counting calories has worked in the past. But modern-day calories have changed because the nutrition contained in a calorie has diminished. The calories that most of us consume are just not the same from a nutritional standpoint as those calories from decades and centuries before. Though it can be argued that a high-calorie diet will cause weight gain and a low-calorie diet will lead to weight-loss, the body's health does not solely rely on this aspect of nutrition. If the body is constantly supplied with calories that have no nutritional value, the body will want to eat more, causing weight gain, obesity and disease.

1925-9: The Lucky Strike cigarette brand launches the "Reach for a Lucky instead of a sweet" campaign, capitalizing on nicotine's appetite-suppressing superpowers. This advertising campaign advised customers to "Reach for a Lucky Instead of a Sweet" and "Light a Lucky and You'll Never Miss Sweets that Make You Fat" was a very successful campaign at the time.

1920 The Hay Diet also known as the **food combining** diet is a nutrition method developed by the New York physician William Howard Hay in the 1920s and became one of the most famous early fad diets. It claims to work by separating food into three groups: alkaline, acidic, and neutral. (Hay's use of these terms does not completely conform to the scientific use, i.e., the pH of the foods.) Acid foods are not combined with the alkaline ones. Acidic foods are protein rich, such as meat, fish, dairy, etc. Alkaline foods are carbohydrate rich, such as rice, grains and potatoes. It has been copied a number of times and Henry Ford followed it.

1930s: Grapefruit Diet
The Grapefruit Diet—a.k.a. the Hollywood Diet—is born. The popular low-cal plan calls for eating grapefruit with every meal and only 800 calories a day.
Of course, it is trotted out every decade or so.

1930: Dr Stoll's Diet Aid and liquid Diets

Sold in beauty salons from 1930 it was the first explicitly designed liquid meal replacement (as distinct from the good old cabbage soup diet) and composed of a teaspoon of chocolate, starch, whole wheat and bran blended in a cup of water for breakfast and lunch. It pioneered the immensely profitable liquid diet industry.

1939: Gaylord Hauser's Eat and Grow Beautiful

Hauser became Hollywood's guru advocating food restrictions, juices, wheat germ, blackstrap molasses, nuts, yogurts and brewer's yeast. Greata Garbo was a client. He dropped his claim to holding a medical degree after he was investigated and was prosecuted by FDA for fraudulent claims but lived a wealthy man in Hollywood to age 89.

1939: The Rice Diet – Duke University

2000cals a day, 5% protein, 3% fat, complex carbs and 150 mg salt as a last chance for hypertense patients with renal failure. 107 of 192 chronically ill patients improved, 25 died and 60 remained the same. The introduction of anti-hypertensive drugs eclipsed it but it still exists in updated versions.

1950s: The Cabbage Soup Diet reemerges and promises you can lose 10–15 pounds in a week by eating a limited diet including cabbage soup every day. Its popularity has continued to the present day, even though, according to observations, "it appears to be nothing more than a recipe for flatulence". Other soup diets have become popular in the decades since, such as the watercress soup diet.

1950s: Mediterranean Diet

The Mediterranean diet has been evolving for more than 5,000 years, with the superior health of the region's inhabitants first noted in a research paper published after World War II. As more research evolved, so did the diet's popularity. It calls for eating little red meat, medium amounts fish and loads of plant -based foods.
Authors Note: This selection of foods has the most evidence for health and what I recommend in Newtrition – The Super-Mediterranean Diet (foods).

1954: The Tapeworm Diet (again)

Urban legend has it that opera singer Maria Callas dropped 65 pounds on the Tapeworm Diet, allegedly by swallowing a parasite-packed pill.

1958: Dr Jarvis 'The Alkaline Diet' (again)

1960: The Zen Macrobiotic Diet

Launched by the Japanese philosopher, George Ohsawa, classing foods into Yin and Yang and claiming, without evidence, to treat cancer such that the AMA and American Cancer Society had to issue a warning that it *"poses a serious hazard to health and is not beneficial in the treatment of cancer"*.

Early 6os: The Vegetable Oil Diet: *Calories Don't Count* was a national bestseller. Obstetrician Dr. Herman Taller's claimed 'eat as much as you want, and wash it down with vegetable oil, via his pill. The FDA later charged Taller with just peddling safflower oil and he was convicted of mail fraud.

1963: Weight Watchers

A self-described "overweight housewife obsessed with cookies" as a young wife in her 20s, Jean Nidetch decided to finally get control of her body, but even after losing 20 pounds in 10 weeks using a diet sponsored by the New York City Board of Health, she found she couldn't seem to stick to the plan in the long term. That was when she realized she needed the support of her friends. Nidetch began holding weekly meetings at her house, passing copies of the Board of Health Diet to anyone who came, with the hope that the more people were dieting together the better they all would do. Bear in mind, this predates the self-help movement and its attendant support-group networks. Nidetch and her friends were making this all up from scratch, and it turned out to be an addictive recipe. Within three months of her first meeting, more than 40 people were cramming into Nidetch's house on a weekly basis. Over the next year, she started several different groups around the New York metro area, finally incorporating her fledgling business in May of 1963. Now down to a trim 142 pounds, Nidetch hosted her first official Weight Watchers meeting, drawing more than 400 attendees.

Authors Note: She is to be congratulated for people, like herself, who need support.

(2010: Jennifer Hudson loses a jaw-dropping 80 pounds on Weight Watchers.
2012: Jessica Simpson loses 60 pounds of baby weight on Weight Watchers).

1964: The Drinking Man's Diet

Was a 50 page paperback by aerial photographer, Robert Cameron, and became a cultural phenomenon and, as a high-protein, low-carb diet paved the way for the Atkins and Dukan Diets. It was criticized by experts but sold 2.4 million copies and is still in print.

1970s: HCG Diet

This diet involves eating around 500 calories a day combined with injections of Human Chorionic Gonadotropin, a hormone taken from pregnant women's urine. HCG is supposed to boost your metabolism to help you lose weight, although the massive calorie restriction is certainly a contributing factor. The diet made headlines in the 70s, and again in 2011.

When I was specializing in London one of my colleagues supplemented his pittance by administering this in Harley Street. I thought it was a con then – and it still is.

1970: The Sleeping Beauty Diet, which involves risky sedation, is rumored to have been tried by Elvis. If so it didn't work.

1970s: Ayds: Were a popular appetite-suppressing candy called but taken off the market in 1980 after the AIDS crisis hit. They were phenylpropanolamine in chocolate, caramel, or butterscotch.

1972: Nutrisystem

Nutrisystem is a weight loss program that home delivers shelf-stable and freeze dried, portion controlled packaged meals. It has helped people achieve short-term weight loss goals but has received criticism from some customers not being able to sustain their weight loss.

1972: The Atkins Diet – Lo-carbs again

The low-carb movement came into full swing with Dr. Robert Atkins "Diet Revolution" book. The eating plan advised limiting carbohydrates to reduce weight as well as the risk of diabetes, high blood pressure and metabolic syndrome. The diet gained new popularity with Atkins' 2002 follow-up, "New Diet Revolutions." Atkins made the controversial argument that the low-carbohydrate diet produces a metabolic advantage because "burning fat takes more calories so you expend more calories". He cited one study in which he estimated this advantage to be 950 Calories (4.0 MJ) per day. A review study published in *Lancet,* concluded that there was no such metabolic advantage and dieters were simply eating fewer calories.

Authors Note: Didn't I tell you?

1975: The Cookie Diet
Florida doctor Sanford Siegal baked up a specially designed diet cookie that's packed with a blend of amino acids. Eating six to nine of these cookies each day, along with sensible meals, was the diet's recipe for losing weight. Hollywood eats it up.

1975: The Stone Age Diet (East African, Inuit and Paleo Diets)
Gastroenterologist, Walter Voegtlin, proposed meats, animal fats and plants but eliminated dairy and grains.

In the 1980s Dr Stanley Eaton published his similar version of the East African diet while others explored the Inuit diet but these "prehistoric diets" took off in 2002 with the Paleo Diet (see below).

1976: The Prolin Diet or Last Chance Diet.
This plan involved foregoing food in favor of drinking a concoction called Prolin created by Robert Linn. It contained hooves, horns, bones and other slaughterhouse by products – but no nutrients. At least 58 people had heart attacks while following this diet, although it was unclear if the attacks were due to fasting, drinking the Prolin or both.

1977: SlimFast
SlimFast started with a shake for breakfast, a shake for lunch and a sensible dinner. The weight loss product line has since grown to include snack bars, protein meal bars and a handful of shake flavors.

1978: The Scarsdale Diet
Dr. Herman Tarnower's "The Complete Scarsdale Medical Diet" outlines a plan for eating carbohydrates, proteins and fats in precise proportions. A jilted girlfriend shot Tarnower two years after the book's publication.

Authors Note: That, or she didn't like the diet restrictions. I am happily married and my wife weights less than 60kg (130lb).

1979: Dexatrim
A diet drug containing phenylpropanolamine (PPA), appears on drugstore shelves. Its formula changes after PPA is linked to an increased risk of stroke in 2000.

1981: The Beverly Hills Diet
The book, published in 1981, showed people how to follow a highly restrictive

six-week food-combining regimen and turned its author, Judy Mazel, into a Hollywood diet "guru" but who had no science or nutritional training. Mazel, clearly inspired by William Hay, believed that the order in which we ate food was the main problem, "confusing" the enzymes in our bodies that digest the food and leading to weight gain. She advocated the eating of rather a lot of "fat-burning" pineapple. For the first 10 days of the diet, only fruit was permitted; gradually other foods were introduced, but protein and carbohydrates were eaten separately. It sold more than a million copies and attracted celebrity fans including Englebert Humperdinck, Linda Gray and Liza Minnelli. Mazel died age aged 63.

1981: The Cambridge Diet

A fad diet in which 600 to 1500 cals are consumed per day, principally in liquids made from commercial products sold as part of the diet regime. These products are manufactured in the UK and include shakes, meal replacement bars, soups and smoothies.

1982: The F Plan

Is a high fiber diet created in the 1980s by British author Audrey Eyton, founder of Slimming Magazine, and based on the work of Denis Burkitt. The *F-Plan diet* book was in the top ten best-selling books in America in April and May 1983. The diet works by restricting the daily intake of calories to less than 1,500 whilst consuming well-above the recommended level of dietary fiber. The fiber has a number of beneficial effects, such as making the dieter feel "full" for much longer than normal, reducing the urge to overeat, and promoting a healthy digestive system. The disadvantages include excessive flatulence in the first few weeks and having to eat food that is harder work to chew and swallow. Some people also express a dislike of the texture of such a high fiber diet. The dieter will need to consume more water than usual to prevent constipation. In 2006 Eyton published "F2", a revised version of the F-plan written in the light of subsequent medical discoveries, which claims to be faster and more effective and campaigns against low-carbohydrate diets, particularly the Atkins Diet.

Authors Note: I am a fan of Dennis Burkitt and high fiber and include this in my Newtrition foods.

1982; The aerobics craze Jane Fonda

Launched her first exercise video, *Workout: Starring Jane Fonda*. Her catch phrase: "No pain, no gain."

Authors Note: Exercise good but unfortunately it only accounts for 15% of weight loss.

1983: Jazzercise
Founded in 1969 by professional dancer Judi Sheppard Missett, hits all USA 50 states.
1983: Jenny Craig
Based on the motto "Eat Well, Move More and Live Life," Jenny Craig is an Australian weight loss and nutrition-based company. Each customized program combines frozen meals and other packaged foods, containing fruits, vegetables, lean meats, as well as meatless options.

1985: Seattle Sutton's Healthy Eating
Illinois registered nurse Seattle Sutton eschewed dietary gimmicks and went for straightforward healthy eating with a plan that delivers well balanced, freshly prepared meals including fresh fruit and vegetables, right to people's doors.
Authors Note: These latter two are sensible and to be recommended
1985: Fit for Life
Written by "nutrition specialists", Harvey and Marilyn Diamond. Prohibits complex carbs and protein from being eaten during the same meal. It lacks any scientific basis, no clinical trials, provokes vitamin, calcium and mineral deficiencies while potentially causing serious complications in diabetics. Nevertheless, it spent 40 weeks on the New York Times Best Seller list and sold over 12 million copies. "Scams sell and science sucks" – especially when it comes to diets.
1985: The Caveman Diet aka "Paleo"

1986: The Rotation Diet
Launched by Martin Katahn, a professor of psychology at Vanderbilt University, involves diet, exercise and behavior modification, it rotates different calorie restrictions over three weeks: 600, 900, 1200 for women and 1.200, 1,500 and 1,800 for men with a period of maintenance. It claims to prevent 'metabolic adaption' as does the Zig-Zag diet

1987: Elizabeth Takes Off
Actress Elizabeth Taylor advises dieters to eat veggies and dip each day at 3 p.m.

1988: Oprah's Liquid Diet
Wearing a pair of size 10 Calvin Klein jeans, Oprah walked onto the set of her show, pulling a wagon full of fat to represent the 67 pounds she lost.

1991: Americans go low-fat
Eating foods like McDonald's McLean Deluxe burger.

1994: The Guide to Nutrition Labeling and Education Act (USA) Requires food companies to include nutritional info on nearly all packaging.

1995: The Zone Diet
Calls for a specific ratio of carbs, fat, and protein at each meal, begins to attract celeb fans.

1997: Blood Type diet.
In Eat Right for Your Type, Peter D'Adamo, a naturopath, claimed that people should eat foods compatible with their blood type. He had no supporting evidence and subsequent studies found "no evidence" and "findings do not support the 'Blood-Type diet hypothesis'".

1997: Stacker 2:
Originally developed for bodybuilders who engaged in the practice of "stacking," or ingesting Ephedrine HCL, caffeine and aspirin for a lean look and extra energy.

2000: Gwyneth Paltrow lends cred to the Macrobiotic Diet, a restrictive Japanese plan based on whole grains and veggies.

2000s: The Dukan diet
A French GP, **Pierre Dukan**. Like the Atkins diet, it involves four stages of weight loss and "stabilization", with the final stage being a diet for life, including eating protein only one day a week.

2002: The Paleo Diet
This high-protein diet by Loren Cordain PhD, includes lean meats, fish, fruit, vegetables and some animal fats, eggs and seeds while avoiding grains, legumes, processed foods, sugar, salt and potatoes. He claimed it was the diet of the Hunter-Gatherer and hence based on our genes. But Cordain was not a medical doctor and humans evolved salivary amylase to digest grains for essential vitamins and legumes have also been found to be nutritionally beneficial – so either Cordain didn't know this or he assumed our ancestors didn't eat grains or legumes - or potatoes – just don't tell the Peruvians or the Irish.

2003: The South Beach Diet
Miami doctor Arthur Agatston, MD, adds fuel to the low-carb craze seen as a more moderate version of Atkins. "No white carbs'.

2004: The Gluten-Free Diet
Gluten free grains have been around forever helping those with coeliac disease, but gluten free diets started gaining widespread popularity around 2004 but have no place in weight control.

2004: Ephedra Ban
The FDA bans the sale of diet drugs and supplements containing ephedra after it's linked to heart attacks.

2004: *The Biggest Loser*
TV debut, turning weight loss into a reality show. All regain weight and their fitness instructor has a heart attack.

2006: Master Cleanse
Beyoncè admits to using the Master Cleanse, a concoction of hot water, lemon juice, maple syrup, and cayenne pepper, to shed 20 pounds for *Dreamgirls*.

2007: Alli
The nonprescription drug is taken with meals to keep your body from absorbing some of the food you eat.

2007: Zantrex
Zantrex weight-loss products have been around since at least 2007, and they're still going strong. Caffeine is one of the main components in their product line.

2009: Whole30 invented by a husband and wife.
Followers are encouraged to eat: Mostly home-cooked meals rich in veggies, meat, eggs, fish, and fruit.

It does not allow: Alcohol, bread (including gluten-free varieties), whole grains, beans, sugar, dairy (including butter), legumes like beans, peanuts, soy, MSG, processed snacks, or "comfort" foods like pancakes or desserts. There's also no weighing yourself allowed during the first month.

Nutritionists are generally critical about the Whole30 regimen. US News and World report consistently puts the plan near the bottom of its annual diet ranking. Whole30 is not backed by science and a month isn't enough time to re-set your digestive system.

2011: The HCG Diet (again)

Combines a fertility drug with a strict 500- to 800-calorie-a-day regimen, invites interest—and criticism.

2012: Fasting Diets

Fasting Diets are as old as God's Dog but with increasing evidence as to their benefit.

Recently popularized on the BBC as the 5:2 diet (eat normally for five days; restrict calories to 500 for women, and 600 for men, on two non-consecutive days), is the current diet trend as – though its supporters would describe it as advice for life rather than a fad diet.

Optavia offers a few different structured weight loss programs – just order a box. While U.S. News & World Report gave it a high ranking for fast weight loss, it did not fare as well for long-term weight loss, nutrition, and heart healthfulness with a lack of fresh food, and highly processed products. It is also expensive

NOTE: Lulu Hunt, The Mediterranean Diet, Weight Watchers, Craig and Sutton prepared meals and Fasting are not Fads or Scams but there is very little that's new – the exception are my list of Super-Foods for which there is modern research for their claims.

And then there's Volumetrics, Flexitarian, Traditional Asian, Slim Fast, SparkPeople, HMR, Flat Belly, Engine 2, South Beach, Abs, Eco-Atkins, Aitkins 40, Macrobiotic, Medifast, Supercharged Hormone, Body Reset, Whole 30, The Mono, Pizza (I kid you not), Wild, Disassociated, Military, The Taco (I kid you not again) and the Golo Diets (to name but a few), they are all scams or don't work.

As you can see from this history ALL diets depend on eating less (or getting a tapeworm to share your food).

Of course, you have to eat less! We all know that!

Losing weight is that simple, according to all these diets, yet it seems the hardest thing possible to achieve. Overweight and obesity, as per the History chapter, have always been a problem but obesity was only recognized as an epidemic in

1985 and coincides with the alteration to our foods, these alterations of processed, ultra-processed, refined and additives, would seem implicated. Especially as they are delicious, cheap and readily available

What are Detox Diets and Cleanses and Does Anyone Need Them?

Whether it's called a detox diet or a cleanse, it doesn't really matter. Neither has a clear-cut definition but both have similar goals -- to rid/cleanse the body of supposedly harmful substances (usually referred to as "toxins").

According to MedlinePlus from the U.S. National Library of Medicine, "Toxins are substances created by plants and animals that are poisonous to humans. Toxins also include some medicines that are helpful in small doses, but poisonous in large amounts. Toxins also include metals, such as lead, and certain chemicals in the environment." However, in the context of commercial detox diets, the meaning of the term "toxin" is often vague or obscure.

In 2009, a group of early career scientists called The Voices of Young Science, created "The Detox Dossier." They went to the manufacturers of 15 representative detox products and asked what toxin their product targeted and what evidence they had to support that claim. They came to the following conclusion:

"No one we contacted was able to provide any evidence for their claims or give a comprehensive definition of what they meant by 'detox'. We concluded that 'detox' as used in product marketing is a myth. Many of the claims about how the body works were wrong and some were even dangerous."

Weight loss is often a secondary goal of detoxes or cleanses. All use a restrictive diet, often in conjunction with a variety of supplements (including herbs, vitamins, seasonings, and so on). For example, The Master Cleanse, also called the Lemonade Diet, is a liquid-only diet consisting of water, lemon juice, maple syrup, and cayenne pepper taken for 10 days. It is essentially a starvation diet. Unfortunately, most of the weight loss in a detox diet is water, and the weight returns just as quickly as it left as soon as a normal diet is resumed.

Detox diets claim that they can help chronic conditions that occur when the body becomes victim to a build-up of "toxins." As Dr. Junger puts it: "When our systems are overtaxed, they begin to break down in a multitude of ways. Allergies, headaches, depression, irritable bowel syndrome, fatigue, weight gain, and insomnia are just a few of the symptoms that can result. The majority of these common ailments are the direct result of toxin build-up in our systems that has accumulated during the course of our daily lives." Dr. Junger's book *Clean* currently is number 7 in Amazon sales rankings for alternative medicine books.

"But the science behind the detox theory is deeply flawed," says Peter Pressman, MD, an internal medicine specialist at Cedars-Sinai Medical Center in Los Angeles. "The body already has multiple systems in place -- including the liver, kidneys, and gastrointestinal tract -- that do a perfectly good job of eliminating toxins from the body within hours of consumption."

Detox dieters often report a variety of benefits, but most of these improvements may be due to changes in the diet unrelated to any change in "toxin levels." For instance, a decrease in headaches could be related to elimination of caffeine or alcohol in the diet. Decreased bloating just from eating less. Clearer skin may be related to better hydration.

Is there any scientific evidence to support the dubious claims of detox proponents? Almost none. There is a 2015 study by Kim et al. "Eighty-four premenopausal women were randomly divided into 3 groups: a control group without diet restriction (Normal-C), a pair-fed placebo diet group (Positive-C), and a lemon detox diet group (Lemon-D). The intervention period was 11 days total: 7 days with the lemon detox juice or the placebo juice, and then 4 days with transitioning food." Women in the Lemon-D and Positive-C groups had significantly greater changes in body weight, BMI, and percentage of body fat than the control group. In addition, serum insulin levels, leptin, and adiponectin levels decreased in the Lemon-D and Positive-C groups. But there was no significant difference between the Lemon-D and Positive-C groups in any of these measurements- suggesting that the main contributing factor was caloric restriction.

A 2015 review by Klein and Kiat, in the *Journal of Human Nutrition and Dietetics*, pointed out a study on UltraClear (Metagenics Inc), the only commercial detox product to have been evaluated clinically. UltraClear is a medical food supplement that purports to detoxify the liver. A study, by MacIntosh and Ball, gave 25 naturopathy students UltraClear for 7 days. There was no placebo control group. They reported a "statistically significant (47%) reduction in the Metabolic Screening Questionnaire [MSQ] scores." The MSQ is a series of questions used to gauge the severity of a variety of health conditions -- from acne, mood swings, and even dark circles under the eyes.

Klein reported that there were (at the time of his review) no current rigorous scientific studies that investigated the effectiveness of commercial detox diets for losing weight.

Are detox diets safe? Possibly, for otherwise healthy people, if used for only a brief period of time. However, the diets can be stressful because of feelings of hunger and deprivation. But prolonged use of these diets can lead to electrolyte imbalances and protein and vitamin deficiencies. Occasionally, there have been reports of potential risks such as kidney damage from green smoothies (Makkapati, 2018) or liver failure from detox teas (Kesavarapu, 2017).

Despite the lack of evidence that detox diets have any real health benefits, they remain incredibly popular due to celebrity endorsements and intensive marketing of the diets and related products. Have any of your patients discussed these diets with you? What has been your reaction or advice?

PERSONALIZED DIETS
Not everybody responds to the same foods in the same way.
The Human Genome Project, completed in 2003, laid the groundwork for scientific research on the environment's influence on gene expression. This led to the increased popularity of nutrigenomics, the field of discovery about how environmental factors, such as food intake and lifestyle impact on us.

It studies the effects of foods and food constituents on gene expression focusing on identifying and understanding molecular-level interaction between nutrients and other dietary bioactives. Peoples' genes can be tested. Gene variants help determine the choice of foods and identifies deficiencies.

Testing can determine for example how quickly you metabolize caffeine, the efficiency with which your body can absorb different vitamins and minerals and even how motivated you are to exercise. But One study showed a nutrigenomic-based diet did not increase weight loss compared to a standard balanced diet. A 2016 meta-analysis found no significant effects of communicating DNA-based risk estimates on diet or physical activity. Another study showed that knowledge of the MTHFR genotype, implicated in the absorption of folate from food, did not significantly improve dietary folate intake. And, although evidence is strong for some gene-diet associations, others remain unclear.

At the present state of knowledge, it is not regarded as good practice to counsel patients to change their diets or lifestyles based on genetics without considering individual clinical biomarkers, dietary and lifestyle preferences and ability to make changes. It may never be possible to prescribe a specific diet based on genetics alone.

Using a nutrigenomic approach has not achieved better results than current nutrition counseling methods.

However, a modified approach is to measure your own blood glucose levels say one then, two hours after a meal.

Some people get significant spikes while others do not, to the *same* food(s)!?

It is thought our gut bacteria, the microbiome, causes this. Good bacteria no spike, bad bacteria – spikes.

You can then either eat the foods that don't cause a spike or alter your microbiome.

As to the latter there is enormous research going into this with many laboratories offering to analyze your microbiome, but I am not sure if any have detailed successful transition methods from bad to good gut bacteria, as yet. So, I would be more inclined to do my own glucose levels and find out what foods, in essence, I don't metabolize well.

But, while we may respond to foods differently and hence be eating the 'wrong' foods and therefore eating the foods which would maximize weight loss, again, all this seems so difficult and complicated.

My fundamental approach is that, as anyone can observe, people who starve lose weight. The corollary, which no one wants to hear, acknowledge or admit to (the Elephant in the room) is that, it is eating more than we need that puts on weight.

K

ADDENDA

CHAPTER 26

ADDENDA

Prevalence
Graph: % of population with BMI >30

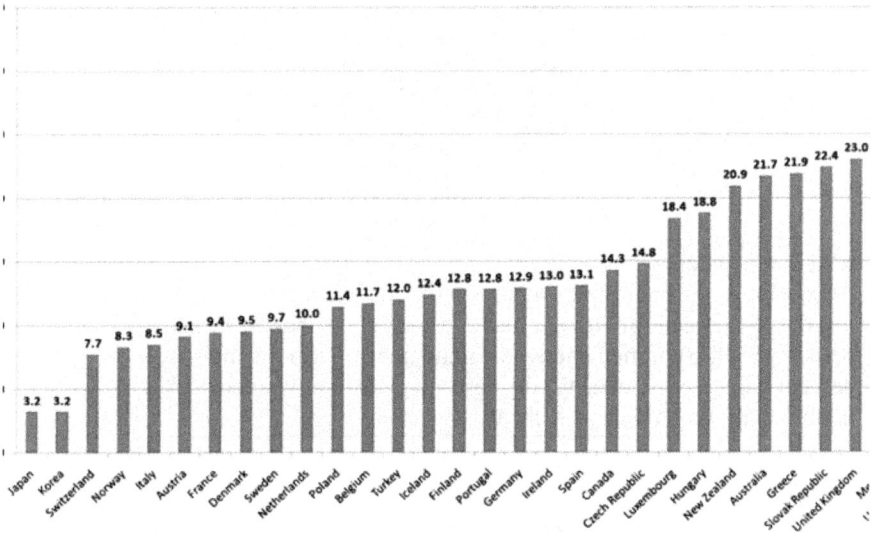

http://diabetescure101.com/BMI.htm,

It is of note that the Japanese are, as a nation, not only the world's leanest but one of the world's longest living. The fact that Japan is the leanest nation with a diet largely of unprocessed seaweed and fish and the USA the fattest on the SAD – Sick American Diet of Super-Sized Processed and fried foods would suggest environment plays a major role in fat gain.

Estimated Percentage by Sex USA

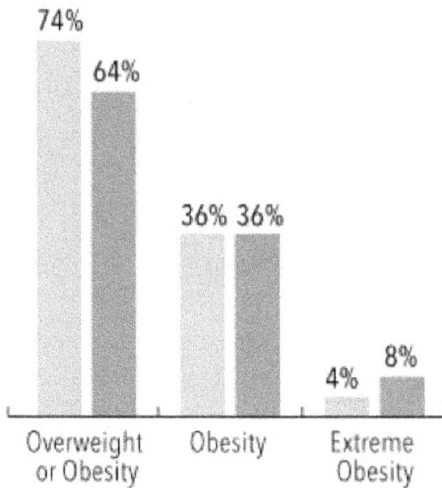

■Men ■ Women

According to the bar graph, 74 percent of men had overweight or obesity; 64 percent of women had overweight or obesity. Equal percentages (36) of men and women had obesity. Among men, 4 percent had extreme obesity; the percentage among women was double that of men, at 8%. NHANES,2009–2010

Fat Kids

We now have the fattest kids in the history of the world and the graph keeps zooming up. Children born since the 1980s are two to three times more likely than older generations to be overweight or obese by the age of 10.[73] 60% of childhood obesity is linked to TV watching and 93% of ads on Kids TV were for junk food.

It is vital, if children are not to be overweight or obese, that parents now become more responsible in as much that they ban sugary drinks and fast foods and promote fruit, nuts and healthy foods as per the Nutrition chapter. The Supermarket aisles are a children's wonderland, an Aladdin's Cave of delicious delights strategically designed and arranged to mesmerize a child into intense desire. No child can be blamed for wanting it, the blame is on the parent for buying it. While it may be easier to give into a screaming child by buying a candy bar it really is tantamount to administering a long-term poison.

[73] PLOS. "UK population is becoming overweight and obese at younger ages." ScienceDaily. ScienceDaily, 19 May 2015. <www.sciencedaily.com/releases/2015/05/150519151302.htm>.

Dental decay was an epidemic in Glasgow in the 1920s due to their 'Sweetie' shops and their addiction to lollies. It is now an epidemic again in the north of England where 30 to 50 % of children aged five years have decay in their teeth due to junk food, sugar and especially sugary drinks. These kids with tooth decay are also invariably overweight or obese. Parents are not educated as to nutrition, often blaming 'glands' or anything else other than their bad diets and lifestyle and are not very responsible such that 1 in 5 children in Leeds miss their specialist dental appointments.[74]

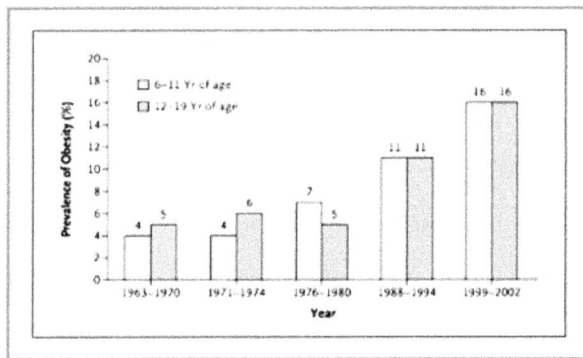

Percentages of U.S. Children and Teenagers Who Were Obese.

It is very rare to find a fat child with thin parents (it is very rare to find a fat dog with thin owners).
90% of obese kids don't lose weight.

More than a third of UK overweight or obese teenagers don't see themselves as being too heavy and think their weight is about right.[75]

---

[74] JUNK FOOD KIDS – Who's To Blame? BBC 2014
[75] S E Jackson, F Johnson, H Croker, J Wardle. Weight perceptions in a population sample of English adolescents: cause for celebration or concern? *International Journal of Obesity*, 2015; DOI: 10.1038/ijo.2015.126

A Complex Problem

Some complexity of the problem of weight, let alone weight loss, can be seen just in the different adiposity spurts between males and females:

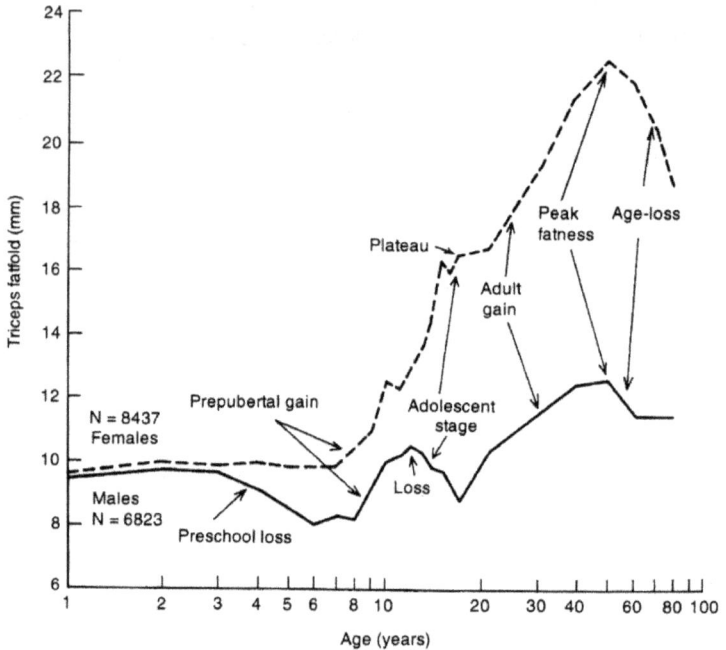

Fig. 7.2 Sex differences in adiposity during adolescence (from: Garn & Clark, 1976). Reproduced with from *Paediatrics* **57** 443–56.

I Don't Care How You Broke Your Leg: Let's Fix It

There is some fascinating research as to why people overeat but your and my concern is not how and why you put on fat but how to get rid of it. It is much harder for some and seemingly impossible for the really obese but blaming your hormones, your stress levels or your genes and now your brain, 'ain't gonna do it'. To put is simply and honestly, you are going to have to eat less (and better). While we are deluged with possible other causes as to obesity, in a study of heart disease which used obese sheep, it was asked, *'How did the researchers create obese sheep?'* The answer was, *'It was easy; they overfed them'*.

When to Start

The American Academy of Pediatrics (AAP) says Obesity Prevention Should Start Before Age 2 beginning with prenatal care. In a clinical report published in *Pediatrics* the group recommends the following:

. Breast-feeding should be encouraged. Pediatricians and obstetricians to promote healthy weight gain during pregnancy.

. Families should have less junk food available in the house (e.g., sugar-sweetened beverages and high-calorie snacks) and make it less prominent. Practically, the cookie jar should be replaced by a fruit bowl.

. Access to televisions and other screens should be limited to 2 hours a day in children over aged 2. Younger children should not have screen time. Televisions should be restricted from children's bedrooms and the kitchen.

. Families should aim for at least 60 minutes of moderate-to-vigorous physical activity every day.

Weight Watchers effective

Treatment by GPs / PCPs have not been very successful.' Modest effectiveness is by referral to evidence based commercial programs. A trial from Australia, Germany and UK assigned participants to standard care national treatment guidelines or 12 months' free membership of Weight Watchers. Those in the commercial group lost an average of 4.1 kg, whereas those in the standard care group lost 1.8 kg. Another trial in England, also suggested that Weight Watchers was more effective than counseling provided in primary care at one year of follow-up. After 12 weeks, average weight loss was 1.4 kg in 70 participants in the primary care group compared with 4.4 kg in the participants in the commercial program.

Eating Less but Gaining Weight

While obesity rates have almost trebled, surprisingly, overall, our actual calorie intake has fallen by around 20% compared to 30 years ago. This would seem impossible, but it can be seen that we are eating different ratios of what we previously ate, eating more junk and processed foods.

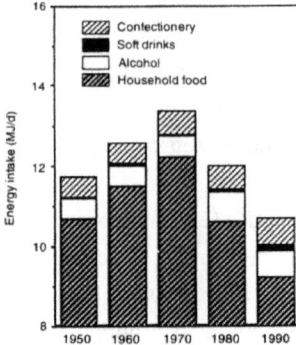

Fig. 13.1 Energy intake including alcohol, soft drinks and confectionery. Data from NFS with additions derived from national supply figures (Prentice & Jebb 1995a).

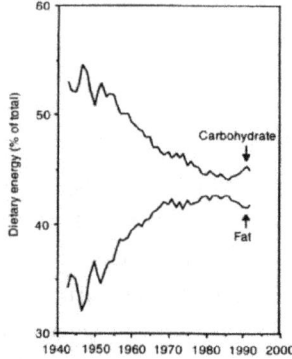

Fig. 13.3 Changes in the proportion of energy derived from fat (data from National Food Survey, Prentice & Jebb 1995a).

This graph shows that while we are eating less in total, *the ratios or composition of the foods we eat have changed,* such that we are eating *relatively* far less 'Household Food', which we can assume is not junk, while, at the same time, our intake of alcohol, processed foods, soft drinks and confectionery has *relatively* increased. We are eating more of the wrong foods which are high in Calories, low in nutrition and which are processed such that we may not metabolize them as efficiently as natural foods.

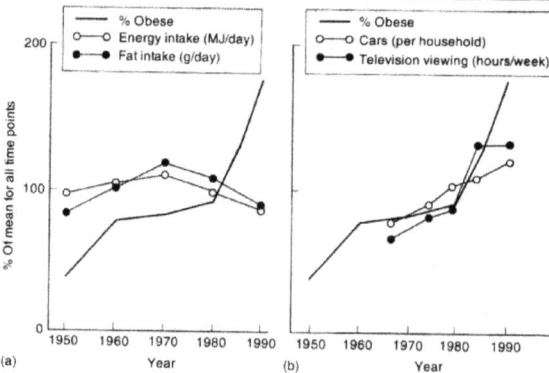

Fig. 15.6 Secular trends in dietary intake (a) and inactivity indicators (b) in relationship to obesity in Britain. The values show percentage for each time point based on an average of 100% timespan (from: Prentice & Jebb, 1995a).

Obesity increases identically to inactivity (Cars & TV)
(Dot lines of eating drop but obesity goes up

Elsewhere it has been pointed out that exercise is not very efficient at losing weight, but these graphs and studies show that obesity increases with inactivity.

A NOTE ON OBESITY

An Editorial in the New England Journal of Medicine claimed that *"the folk belief that overeating causes obesity...has two fatal flaws"*: 1) is that only if one is fat can one be said to have over-eaten and 2) in well-designed experiments eating behavior has been shown to be the dependent (stable) variable rather than the independent (changing) variable.[76] In other words obese people only ate fixed amounts and there were other causes to their weight gain.

The recent concept is that obesity is a multifactorial disease including medical (genetic, endocrine), environmental conditions (24hr lifestyle, economics, global stressors), micro-environmental influences (eating schedules, physical activity, sleep patterns, drugs) with the ultimate consequence being failure of the homeostasis of weight and energy regulatory mechanisms, leading to an elevated body fat set point.

The AMA classified obesity as a disease in 2013.

But obesity in the USA in the 1960s and 1970s was only 13% of U.S. adults; by 1990 it was only 15%, by 2010 it was 25%, today it is 40%.

Are these obesity gurus, as above, seriously trying to tell me eating in these people has not increased or more's the point, a new disease has developed consequent to their microbiome and gene changes?

Axs a panel of obesity experts concluded in 2018: "The prevalence of obesity has increased so rapidly that the causes of the epidemic have to be environmental rather than genetic- genetically regulated changes would take much, much longer to manifest.
That is not to say there are no genetic associations, there are, but they are responsible for a relatively small percentage of the obesity prevalence observed".[77]

And this is obesity, not just overweight which combined accounts for now over 70% of most Western countries.

My take on this is that there are people who absorb more calories and lay down

---

[76] NEJM- March 9, 1995 – Vol. 332, No 10.
[77] Practical Challenges in Obesity. Medscape 26 Sep 2018.

fat more easily than others. Incredibly so. This leads to morbid obesity and is a profound medical problem beyond the advice in this, Slim 4 Life Program, which is for those of us who have become overweight by insidiously eating more – it only takes 20cals a day and I maintain that, to put on fat *you still have to have eaten the calories to begin with*. And, despite these "well-designed experiments" obesity has only been an epidemic since the 1980s and there are daily *practical*, rather than experimental, studies and trials, wherein it is recorded that in the USA they are eating 788 *extra* calories a day, and are eating altered, processed food which coincides with this new, previously unknown epidemic.

Go figure.

RESUME: BED
Behavior, Exercise, Diet

A. **RECOMMENDED DIETS** (select one to suit)
1. Reduce all meals every day (ED) by a minimum 10% up to 25%.
2. Do Intermittent Fasting (IF) (500 - 600 calories) two days a week
3. 16:8 Eat for 8 hours fast for 16 hours (no breakfast)

B. **COMMIT**: DETERMINATION, DEDICATION, DISCIPLINE, RESOLVE, RESTRAINT

C. **NEWTRITION**: High quality. No processed or prepared foods.

D. **EXERCISE**:
SIT: 20 seconds x2 (40 secs in toto), x3 times a week
Resistance Training: one area once a week

E. **SUPERVISION & ENCOURAGEMENT** – Smartphone App
- Plan Ahead

F. **BREAK HABITS** – Do Something Different (DSD)

G. **DISILLUSIONMENT**: Plan
- Re-list the reasons you want to lose
- Realistic goals 250g/wk
- Look at this list: Read this book
- Reorganize your plan, start again, get help
- Enjoy gaining control and getting fit
- Be Positive: You may not be losing but getting fit

H. **NOT LOSING**
- Intake wrongly estimated – get monitored
- Default value hit – keep going – break through
- You cannot lose every week. Keep going
- No unreal expectations: Weight loss is s-l-o-w
- Ideal loss is 250g a week (that's 13kg a year!)
- Premenstrual water retention
- Enjoy gaining control and getting fit.
- Don't be discouraged by setbacks. Push through

- Learn to read labels. 'Sugar' is disguised as alternate names
- Simplest is to avoid all packaged or wrapped food
- Mother Hubbard (bare cupboard): Don't buy it you can't eat it
- No fat patient thinks they eat to excess. Their satiety index is set high
- They honestly don't know they are eating more than they need
- There was never a fat prisoner of war but our genes or our microbiome haven't changed
- Fat owners have fat dogs
- Eating less is 85% of weight loss, 15% is exercise
- But you need BOTH!
- The exercise needed to burn off food calories is far too great to correlate with actual weight lost. There must be some other mechanism at work especially with Resistance Weight Training
- Exercise make you *more efficient at metabolizing* food and burning off Calories and it also reduces mortality
- But you can eat smarter: Women who ate more fruit and vegetables which were water-rich, lost 33% more weight in the first 6 months compared to those on a low-fat diet. Despite the fact they ate more food by weight, they actually ate less Calories
- Eat high volume, high nutrition. Water content is the key

I. **MAINTENANCE MONITORING**

1. Are meals smaller?
2. Are you leaving some food on your plate
3. Do you stop before you feel full
4. Non-hungry eating?
5. 'Mindless snacks': More formal meals
6. Weigh daily
7. Are there less fat and refined carbohydrates
8. Is exercise > 30 mins a day or SIT
9. Look up daily Calorie needs for age, height and sex and don't exceed – in fact eat 600 cals less
10. Although weight loss is achievable for many adults, weight maintenance is elusive

KEY ESSENTIALS

1. Commit- Make Time - Resolve
2. Phone App – record *everything* - 10% loss
3. Chew slowly – up to 42% loss
4. Wait 20 minutes to abate hunger
5. Eat less. Select diet that works for you
6. No snacks after dinner
7. Discard all processed foods. Avoid eating any

1. Newtrition Super-Mediterranean Foods
2. Plan Ahead
3. Identify Triggers
4. Change bad Habits for better Lifestyles
5. Weigh daily
6. Smaller portions / plates
7. Any gain then starve next day until lost
8. Put up a photo of a shape you'd like to be
9. Fruit bowl only on kitchen bench
10. 40 seconds three times a week exercise bike
11. Resistance training
12. Don't eat more because you exercise
13. Water boarding. Hi-volume, lo-cal foods
14. Take the stairs
15. Waists: Men < 102 cm. Women < 88 cm

Snacks – foods that fill more[78]

i.	Potatoes	ix.	Grapes
ii.	White fish	x.	Bread
iii.	Porridge		wholemeal
iv.	Oranges	xi.	Popcorn
v.	Apples	xii.	All Bran
vi.	Pasta brown	xiii.	Eggs
vii.	Beef steak	xiv.	Cheese
viii.	Baked Beans	xv.	Rice white
xvi.	Lentils		

Slim 4 Life advice is for chilled grapes or apples and potatoes if cold
Foods with high water content: Fill you more with less calories
Cucumbers and iceberg lettuce 96% water.
Celery, tomatoes and zucchini: 95-94% water
Broccoli, cabbage, cauliflower, capsicums, spinach: 93-91% water

Finally, it has been observed that 'the price of freedom is eternal vigilance'.

This too, is the price of keeping ourselves slim and trim.

---

[78] These are based on a Sydney University study done in the 1990s where white bread was rated as 100 at 24th.

FOOD USED TO BE SCARCE AND NATURAL

AND

WE HAD TO WALK, EVEN RUN!

NOW FOOD IS IN OVERSUPPLY AND UNNATURAL

AND

WE SIT AT WORK, IN OUR CARS AND WATCH TV

AND

WE ARE THE FATTEST RACE IN HISTORY

GO FIGURE

EPILOGUE

One of my patients is a lean Consultant Anesthetist whose slimness I have admired over a decade or so. I thought he had the 'slim gene' even though I did note that on one visit he had walked some seven kilometers from his hospital to my branch surgery (and back again). He was kindly complementing me on my Newtrition book and I told him how I was now finishing this 'Slim 4 Life' book, adding that 'he didn't need it as he had the slim gene' but for the rest of us we had to strive to eat less.

He soon put me in my place. He told me how hard he works at keeping trim and how every day he has to resist food and finds it tough.

Driving home that night I recounted this story to my (trim) wife pointing out how even those people we may erroneously think that it is easy for them as being 'naturally slim', still have to work at it.

I was in for yet another surprise revelation.

She then informed me, just as firmly as my anesthetist colleague, that she too had to work very hard at staying slim and how 'she would never be fat' and how "If I put on two kilos that's it! I don't eat until I've lost it".

After 35 years I was startled that I never knew this about her.

So both of these, what I had considered 'naturally' slim people, in fact, worked daily, quietly and very hard at being slim.

A lesson for us all I think.

There's that word "restraint" again.

All the weight books seem to boast how their authors lost so much weight. For the record I have lost 18kg over a decade which I put on, not through junk food, but pure un-thinking, over-indulgence.

Two kilos,
That's it!
Gotta stop eating,
Gotta get fit.

INDEX

A
Abdominal obesity 172
Accelerometers 136
Advertising 85, 156, 159
Alcohol 105
Alternate Regimes Swiss 10
Amylase 121
Assertion 87
Attitude 67
Avoidance 86

B
Behaviour Modification 47
BED 51
Berri berri 122
Biggest Losers 97
Binges 98
Body Shapes 61
Blame 100
BMI ix
Boredom 101
Breakfast Cereal racket 154
Breakfast - World's best 116
Browns University National Registry 12
Bundling 157
Bus vs car 145

C
Calories needed to gain weight 22
Calorific needs 7
Calorie Restriction and Health 171
Calorie restriction and longevity 169
Carbohydrates 40
    Refined 125

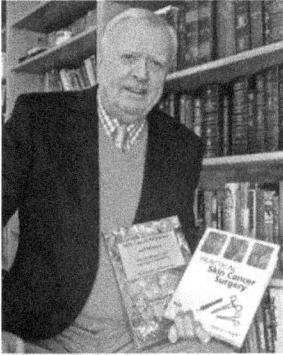

Mileham Hayes graduated in medicine from the University of Queensland then specialised in Sydney, Edinburgh and London being elevated to a Fellow of both Royal Colleges of Physicians.

He was appointed to the world's first Coronary Care Unit where his interest in Preventive Medicine was stimulated as Cardio Vascular Disease was, and is, our greatest killer and which can be prevented by good nutrition and weight control (hence this book). He had also inherited the shrewd observations of his Father which were ahead of his time as to good nutrition and the damage smoking causes.

In Edinburgh he was attached to, what must have been, one of the world's first Obesity Units and weight control has been an on-going study, culminating in Slim 4 Life as, for the past 50 years of treating patients, he has had to witness the failures of the never ending repetition of diet fads and scams.

He was awarded the Order of Australia in 1996.

Slim 4 Life differs in that it is based on the best medical trials and evidence and provides a complete program because diets are not enough.

www.ingramcontent.com/pod-product-compliance
Lightning Source LLC
Chambersburg PA
CBHW070921030426
42336CB00014BA/2482